The Herbal Remedies
&
Natural Medicine Bible

(5 in 1)

Discover 50 Organic Homemade Teas & Medicinal Recipes to Solve Common Ailments, Detox Your Body, and Improve Your Health & Wellbeing

Laya M. Barry

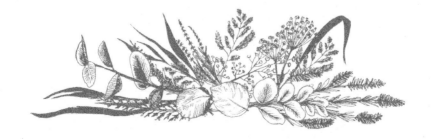

Contents

Introduction

Plants and herbs are an essential part of human life, providing a range of benefits that have been recognized for centuries. They are used for medicinal purposes, culinary purposes, and even as decoration in homes and gardens. The use of plants and herbs dates back to ancient times, when they were used for religious, medicinal, and ceremonial purposes. Plants and herbs have been utilized for their medicinal properties throughout history. The ancient Egyptians used plants such as aloe vera and garlic for their healing properties. In traditional Chinese medicine, herbs such as ginseng and licorice root have been used for thousands of years to treat a variety of ailments. Similarly, in Ayurvedic medicine, which originated in India, herbs such as turmeric and holy basil are used to promote health and wellness.

In addition to their medicinal uses, plants, and herbs are also widely used for culinary purposes. Herbs such as basil, oregano, and rosemary are commonly used to add flavor to dishes, while plants such as garlic and onions are used to enhance the taste of food. Tea, which is made from herbs such as chamomile and peppermint, is also a popular beverage consumed around the world. Plants and herbs are not only used for their medicinal and culinary benefits but also for their aesthetic properties. Flowers such as roses and lilies are used for decoration in homes and gardens, while plants such as ferns and succulents are used for their visual appeal and ability to purify the air.

Today, the use of plants and herbs has become more widespread, with a growing interest in natural and alternative medicines. People are looking for natural remedies that can help improve their overall health and well-being without the negative side effects often associated with traditional medicines. The global market for herbal and plant-based products has also grown significantly in recent years, with the market projected to reach USD 86.74 billion by 2026. This growth is attributed to a variety of factors, including the increasing prevalence of chronic diseases, a growing interest in natural and organic products, and a rising awareness of the potential health benefits of plants and herbs. The use of plants and herbs is not without its challenges.

One of the most significant challenges is the need for proper regulation and quality control. Due to the lack of standardized regulations and quality control procedures, the

safety and efficacy of herbal products can vary greatly. This has led to concerns regarding the potential risks associated with the use of these products. Another challenge is the sustainability of the plant and herb industry. The increasing demand for these products has led to overharvesting and depletion of some species, which can have a significant impact on the environment and local communities.

Chapter 1
PLANTS AND HERBS

PECULIARITIES OF HERBS AND PLANTS IN THE WORLD

Plants and herbs are an essential part of the natural world, playing a vital role in the ecosystem, and providing many benefits to humans. With over 300,000 species of plants known to exist, each with its unique characteristics and uses, there is a vast diversity of plants and herbs worldwide. Here are some of the peculiarities of plants and herbs in the world.

- **Adaptation to Different Environments:** Plants and herbs have adapted to different environments and conditions to survive, and some can thrive in the most extreme environments. For instance, cactus plants can survive in hot and dry conditions with minimal water, while Venus's flytraps thrive in nutrient-poor soil, and some plants can survive in salty soil. These adaptations have allowed plants and herbs to grow and thrive in various parts of the world.

- **Medicinal Properties:** Many plants and herbs have medicinal properties, which have been used for centuries to treat various ailments. For example, ginger is known to help with nausea and vomiting, while chamomile is used to promote relaxation and sleep. Other herbs, such as echinacea, have been used to boost the immune system, and garlic is believed to help with cardiovascular health.

- **Culinary Uses:** Plants and herbs are commonly used in cooking to add flavor and nutrition to dishes. Some herbs, such as basil, thyme, and rosemary, are used to season meats and vegetables, while others, such as parsley, are used to garnish dishes. Spices such as cinnamon and nutmeg are also used in cooking and baking.

- **Aesthetic Value:** Plants and herbs are also valued for their aesthetic qualities, with many people enjoying gardens and natural settings filled with colorful flowers, lush greenery, and fragrant herbs. Plants and herbs are also used for landscaping and to decorate indoor spaces.

- **Ecological Importance:** Plants and herbs play a crucial role in the ecosystem, producing oxygen and absorbing carbon dioxide, which helps to reduce the effects of climate change. They also provide habitats and food for various animal species, contributing to biodiversity.

Summarily, the peculiarities of plants and herbs in the world are diverse and unique. From their adaptations to different environments, medicinal properties, culinary uses, aesthetic value, and ecological importance, plants and herbs play a vital role in the natural world and contribute to human health and wellbeing.

PLANTS AND HERBS – SORTED ALPHABETICALLY

There are countless herbs and plants in the world, each with its own unique characteristics and peculiarities. Here are 20 herbs and plants from around the world sorted alphabetically.

- ***ALOE VERA***

Aloe vera is a succulent plant with calming and hydrating properties. It originated in Africa but is now cultivated in tropical and subtropical climates worldwide. The plant can reach a maximum height of 3 feet and has dense, fleshy leaves with serrated margins.

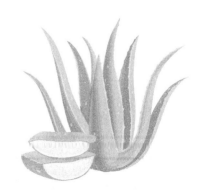

__USES:__ Aloe vera is extensively utilized for its medicinal and cosmetic benefits. It is frequently found in lotions and cosmetics because it is effective at treating sunburns, dry skin, and other skin irritations. Aloe vera is also used to promote healthy digestion

and treat constipation in digestive supplements. Additionally, aloe vera's potential anti-inflammatory, antioxidant, and antibacterial properties have been investigated.

HABITATS: Aloe vera is a robust plant that can thrive in a variety of environments, such as deserts, forests, and grasslands. It requires little water and can tolerate intense heat and sunlight. Aloe vera is commonly found in tropical and subtropical regions, such as Africa, Asia, and Latin America.

ACTIVE PRINCIPLES: The substance within the Aloe vera plant contains a number of active ingredients, such as polysaccharides, anthraquinones, and glycoproteins. Long chains of sugar molecules called polysaccharides are believed to have anti-inflammatory properties. Anthraquinones are compounds with a cathartic effect that are frequently found in digestive aids. Glycoproteins are compounds that have anti-inflammatory and moisturizing properties on the skin.

EFFECTS AND CONTRADICATIONS: There are some potential adverse effects and contraindications to be aware of, despite the fact that aloe vera is generally regarded as safe. When applied topically, aloe vera may cause skin irritation or allergic reactions in some individuals. In addition, aloe vera is a natural laxative and should not be consumed in excessive quantities, as it may cause diarrhea or abdominal discomfort.

TRADITIONAL USES: Aloe vera has been utilized for thousands of years due to its medicinal properties. In traditional African and Ayurvedic medicine, aloe vera was used to treat a variety of conditions, such as constipation, skin irritations, and digestive problems. Aloe vera was also utilized by the ancient Egyptians for its medicinal properties, as it was believed to have anti- inflammatory and wound-healing properties. In many parts of the globe, aloe vera is still used in traditional medicine and is also widely used in modern medicine and cosmetics.

- **ALFALFA**

USES: Alfalfa is commonly used as a dietary supplement due to its high nutritional content. It is believed to support digestive health, alleviate menopausal symptoms, promote liver health, and boost immunity.

HABITATS: Alfalfa is native to Southwest Asia and is now cultivated in various parts of the world, including North America and Europe.

ACTIVE PRINCIPLES: *Alfalfa contains vitamins (A, C, and K), minerals (calcium, iron, and potassium), phytoestrogens, and antioxidants.*

EFFECTS AND CONTRAINDICATIONS: *Alfalfa is generally safe when consumed as food or taken in recommended doses as a supplement. However, it may interact with certain medications, so it's advisable to consult a healthcare professional before using it.*

TRADITIONAL USES: *Traditional herbal medicine uses alfalfa for its diuretic, antidiabetic, and anti-inflammatory properties.*

- **BASIL**

Basil (Ocimum basilicum) is a fragrant herb native to Central Africa and Southeast Asia. It is a popular herb used in numerous dishes around the globe, including pasta sauces, salads, and soups. Basil has a history of medicinal use in addition to its culinary applications.

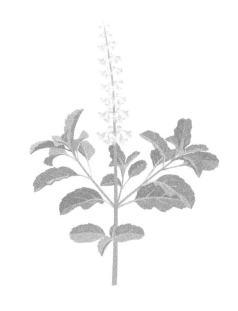

USES: *Basil has antibacterial, antiviral, and anti-inflammatory properties. It is also abundant in antioxidants, which aid in protecting the body from oxidative stress and inflammation. Basil is frequently used to treat digestive issues, including bloating, flatulence, and gastric cramps. In addition, it is used to alleviate tension and anxiety, promote sleep, and treat respiratory conditions like coughs and asthma. Basil oil is frequently used in aromatherapy to induce relaxation and reduce tension.*

HABITATS: *Basil thrives in warm, sunny climates and can be found in gardens, fields, and pastures all over the globe. It thrives best in well-drained soil and requires consistent irrigation. Basil is an annual plant, which means its life cycle is completed in one growing season and it must be replanted annually.*

ACTIVE PRINCIPLES: *Basil contains numerous active compounds, such as essential oils, flavonoids, and phenolic acids. Basil's essential oils are abundant in eugenol, linalool, and citronellol, which are responsible for its distinctive aroma and many of its therapeutic properties.*

EFFECTS AND CONTRADICATIONS: *Basil is generally regarded as safe when ingested in food or as a dietary supplement in the amounts recommended. However, excessive basil consumption can cause digestive distress and, in uncommon cases, allergic reactions. Basil oil should be utilized with caution, as it is highly concentrated and potentially poisonous if consumed in large quantities. As basil oil can stimulate uterine contractions, pregnant women should also avoid using it.*

TRADITIONS USES: *Basil has been used in Ayurvedic, Chinese, and Western herbal medicine for centuries. It has been used to treat a variety of conditions, including digestive problems, respiratory infections, and stress-related disorders. Basil is used in Ayurvedic medicine to treat respiratory ailments and digestive issues and to promote mental clarity and concentration. Basil is used in Chinese medicine to alleviate tension and promote relaxation, as well as to treat digestive issues and respiratory infections. Basil is commonly used in Western herbal medicine to relieve digestive distress and promote relaxation.*

- **BAY LEAVES**

USES: *Bay leaves are commonly used as a culinary herb to add flavor to various dishes. They are also used in traditional medicine for their potential antibacterial, antifungal, and antioxidant properties.*

HABITATS: *Bay leaves come from the bay laurel tree, native to the Mediterranean region, and are now cultivated in many parts of the world.*

ACTIVE PRINCIPLES: *Bay leaves contain essential oils (such as eucalyptol, cineol, and pinene), tannins, and flavonoids.*

EFFECTS AND CONTRAINDICATIONS: *When used in culinary amounts, bay leaves are generally safe. However, consuming large amounts or eating whole leaves can pose a choking hazard. People with allergies to plants in the Lauraceae family should avoid bay leaves.*

TRADITIONAL USES: *Traditional uses of bay leaves include aiding digestion, relieving respiratory issues, and reducing inflammation.*

- ## *CALENDULA*

USES: *Calendula, also known as marigold, is commonly used topically in skincare products and herbal ointments for its soothing and healing properties. It may help with skin conditions, minor wounds, and inflammation.*

HABITATS: *Calendula is native to Europe and parts of Asia but is now cultivated worldwide.*

ACTIVE PRINCIPLES: *Calendula contains flavonoids, triterpenoids, carotenoids, and essential oils.*

EFFECTS AND CONTRAINDICATIONS: *Calendula is generally well-tolerated when used topically. Some individuals may experience skin irritation or allergic reactions. It is not recommended for internal use during pregnancy or breastfeeding without consulting a healthcare professional.*

TRADITIONAL USES: *Traditional uses of calendula include wound healing, soothing skin irritations, and relieving menstrual discomfort.*

- ## *CHAMOMILE*

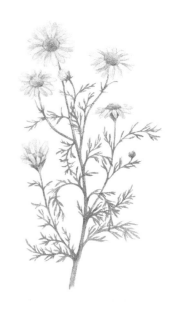

Chamomile has been utilized for centuries due to its medicinal properties. It is typically ingested as a tea and is renowned for its calming and relaxing properties. This article provides a comprehensive summary of chamomile, including its uses, habitats, active principles, effects, contraindications, and traditional applications.

USES: *Chamomile is used for a variety of reasons, including its soothing and relaxing effects, benefits for digestive health, and anti-inflammatory properties. It is frequently employed as a natural remedy for anxiety and stress, and it may also enhance sleep quality. Chamomile is also well-known for its ability to assist digestion and alleviate gastrointestinal issues such as bloating, cramping, and nausea. In addition, chamomile possesses anti-inflammatory and antioxidant properties, making it a possible natural treatment for skin irritations and infections.*

HABITATS: *Chamomile is native to Europe and Western Asia but is now widely distributed throughout the globe. It grows in a variety of environments, including fields, meadows, and gardens, and prefers well-drained soil and full sunlight.*

ACTIVE PRINCIPLES: *In addition to flavonoids, terpenoids, and coumarins, chamomile also contains a number of other medicinally active compounds. These substances possess anti-inflammatory, antioxidant, and sedative properties.*

EFFECTS AND CONTRADICATIONS: *While chamomile is generally considered safe for most individuals, it can cause adverse effects in some. It is possible for allergic reactions to occur, particularly in those who are allergic to ragweed and other members of the Asteraceae family. Additionally, chamomile may interact with certain medications, such as blood thinners and sedatives. Before using chamomile as a natural remedy, it is essential to consult a healthcare professional.*

TRADITIONAL USES: *Chamomile has been utilized for its medicinal properties for centuries. In traditional medicine, it has been used to alleviate anxiety, insomnia, and digestive disorders, among others. Additionally, it has been used topically to treat skin irritations like eczema and psoriasis. Chamomile is used as a natural remedy for menstrual cramping and other women's health issues in some cultures.*

- **DAMIANA**

USES: *Damiana is often used as an herbal supplement to support relaxation, boost mood, enhance libido, and promote overall well-being. It is also used as a flavoring agent in some herbal teas.*

HABITATS: *Damiana is native to Central America, Mexico, and the Caribbean, and is now cultivated in various regions around the world.*

ACTIVE PRINCIPLES: *Damiana contains flavonoids, terpenes, and essential oils.*

EFFECTS AND CONTRAINDICATIONS: *Damiana is generally considered safe when used in recommended amounts. However, it may interact with certain medications or have stimulating effects. It is not recommended for use during pregnancy or breastfeeding.*

TRADITIONAL USES: *Traditionally, damiana has been used as an aphrodisiac, nerve tonic, and digestive aid.*

- ***DANDELION***

USES: *Dandelion is a versatile herb used for various purposes. It is often used as a diuretic, digestive aid, and liver tonic. It is also consumed as a leafy green vegetable and used in herbal teas and dietary supplements.*

HABITATS: *Dandelion is a common plant found in temperate regions throughout the world. It grows in lawns, meadows, and other grassy areas.*

ACTIVE PRINCIPLES: *Dandelion contains vitamins (A, C, and K), minerals (potassium, calcium, and iron), flavonoids, and bitter compounds called sesquiterpene lactones.*

EFFECTS AND CONTRAINDICATIONS: *Dandelion is generally considered safe for most people when consumed in moderate amounts. However, individuals with an allergy to plants in the Asteraceae family or certain medical conditions should exercise caution. Dandelion may interact with certain medications, so it's advisable to consult a healthcare professional if you have specific concerns.*

TRADITIONAL USES: *Traditional uses of dandelion include supporting liver health, promoting digestion, and acting as a natural diuretic.*

- ***ECHINACEA***

Echinacea, also known as purple coneflower, is native to North America. Native American communities have utilized it for centuries due to its medicinal properties. Today, echinacea is extensively used for its immune-boosting properties and is available in capsules, extracts, and teas, among other forms.

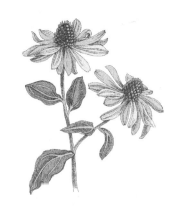

USES: *Echinacea is used to strengthen the immune system and prevent or treat respiratory infections. It is believed to stimulate the production of white blood cells, which aid the immune system in combating infections. Additionally, echinacea is used to treat urinary tract infections, ear infections, and cutaneous infections.*

HABITATS: *Echinacea is indigenous to North America and grows in prairies, meadows, and arid, open woodlands. This plant can withstand a wide spectrum of temperatures and soil conditions.*

ACTIVE PRINCIPLES: *Echinacea contains numerous active compounds such as echinacosides, polysaccharides, and alkamides. It is believed that these compounds are responsible for echinacea's immune-boosting properties. Echinacea contains flavonoids, which have anti-inflammatory and antioxidant properties.*

EFFECTS AND CONTRADICATIONS: *When taken as directed, echinacea is generally considered safe for most individuals. Nonetheless, some individuals may experience adverse effects, including nausea, stomach pain, and dizziness. People with autoimmune disorders such as lupus or rheumatoid arthritis should not use echinacea because it may stimulate the immune system and exacerbate symptoms. People with allergies to plants in the daisy family should also avoid echinacea, as it may cause an allergic reaction.*

TRADITIONAL USES: *Native American communities have historically utilized echinacea for its medicinal properties. It was used to treat numerous ailments, including toothaches, sore throats, and snake stings. In the 1800s, European settlers in North America began using echinacea to treat colds and influenza.*

- **FENNEL**

USES: *Fennel is commonly used as a culinary herb and a medicinal plant. It is known for its digestive properties and is used to relieve bloating, gas, and indigestion. Fennel seeds are also used to make herbal tea, which can help alleviate menstrual cramps.*

HABITATS: *Fennel is native to the Mediterranean region but is now grown worldwide. It thrives in sunny locations and can be found in fields, gardens, and along roadsides.*

ACTIVE PRINCIPLES: *Fennel contains essential oils, including anethole, which is responsible for its characteristic aroma and flavor. It also contains flavonoids and antioxidants.*

EFFECTS AND CONTRAINDICATIONS: *Fennel is generally safe for most people when consumed in moderate amounts as a spice or herbal tea. However, some individuals may experience allergic reactions or skin sensitivity. It may also have estrogenic effects and should be used with caution by individuals with estrogen-sensitive conditions.*

TRADITIONAL USES: *Fennel has been used traditionally to support digestion, improve lactation in breastfeeding mothers, and promote menstrual health. It has also been used for its diuretic properties and as a natural breath freshener.*

• GARLIC

Garlic is a pungent herb (Allium sativum) that has been used for medicinal and culinary purposes for centuries. It is cultivated in many regions of the world, including Asia, Europe, and North America, and is a member of the onion family.

USES: *Garlic is frequently used to give flavor to food, but it is also well-known for its numerous health benefits. It contains sulfur compounds, which account for its distinctive odor and many of its therapeutic properties. It has been demonstrated that these compounds possess antioxidant, anti-inflammatory, and antimicrobial properties. Garlic is frequently used to treat numerous health conditions, such as high blood pressure, excessive cholesterol, and the common cold.*

HABITATS: *Garlic is a hardy herb that can thrive in gardens, fields, and forests, among other environments. It prefers well-drained soil and full exposure for optimal growth. Garlic is typically grown as an annual crop and can be harvested when the leaves begin to turn yellow in the autumn.*

ACTIVE PRINCIPLES: *Allicin, alliin, and ajoene are sulfur-based active ingredients found in garlic. These compounds are responsible for many of the medicinal effects of garlic. Garlic also contains flavonoids and polysaccharides, as well as vitamins and minerals such as vitamin C and selenium.*

EFFECTS AND CONTRAINDICATIONS: *In moderate quantities, garlic is generally considered safe for consumption by the majority of individuals. Garlic can induce gastrointestinal distress in high doses, including nausea, vomiting, and diarrhea. Garlic may also interact with certain medications, including blood-thinning medications; therefore, it is essential to consult a healthcare provider prior to taking garlic supplements. Garlic allergies can cause symptoms such as hives, irritation, and difficulty breathing in some individuals. Those who are allergic to garlic should avoid consuming it.*

TRADITIONAL USES: *For millennia, garlic has been used for medicinal purposes. Garlic was utilized by the ancient Egyptians, Greeks, and Romans for its health benefits. Garlic is utilized in traditional Chinese medicine to treat a variety of maladies, including coughs, colds, and stomach problems. Garlic is* used in Ayurvedic medicine to treat digestive issues and strengthen the immune system. Garlic has been shown to have numerous health benefits in recent times. It has been shown to lower blood pressure, decrease cholesterol levels, and enhance immune function. Garlic is believed to have anti-cancer properties and may aid in the prevention of certain types of cancer.

- **GINGER**

Ginger (Zingiber officinale) is a flowering plant whose medicinal and culinary properties are extensively utilized. Native to Southeast Asia, it is now cultivated in many tropical regions worldwide. Ginger's peppery and pungent flavor makes it a popular ingredient in a variety of foods and beverages.

USES: Ginger has numerous medicinal and culinary applications. It is frequently used to treat digestive problems like nausea, regurgitation, and bloating. Additionally, ginger is used to reduce inflammation, alleviate pain, and strengthen the immune system. Moreover, ginger is frequently used as a flavoring agent in cooking and baking, particularly in Asian cuisine.

HABITATS: Ginger flourishes in warm, humid environments and is typically cultivated in tropical regions. It is frequently cultivated in India, China, and Indonesia, as well as in certain regions of Africa and South America.

ACTIVE PRINCIPLES: Ginger's active components, gingerols, and shogaols, are responsible for its medicinal properties. These substances possess anti-inflammatory, analgesic, and antiemetic properties. In addition to these compounds, ginger also contains zingerone and beta-carotene.

EFFECTS AND CONTRADICATIONS: Ginger is generally harmless for the majority of individuals when consumed in moderation. However, ginger in high doses can induce digestive problems such as heartburn and diarrhea. Ginger may also interact with certain medications, such as blood thinners, so it is essential to consult a healthcare provider before consuming significant quantities of ginger.

TRADITIONAL USES: Ginger has been utilized as a remedy for centuries, particularly in traditional Chinese and Ayurvedic medicine. Ginger is believed to stimulate the circulation of qi (energy) in the body and is used to treat a variety of maladies, including colds, coughs, and menstrual cramps, according to Chinese medicine. Ginger is used to treat digestive issues and is believed to have a warming effect on the body in Ayurvedic medicine.

- ***GINSENG***

Ginseng is a perennial herb that has been used for thousands of years for its medicinal properties. It is native to North America and Asia and is a member of the Araliaceae family. Ginseng's therapeutic effects are attributed to its active compounds, which are known as ginsenosides.

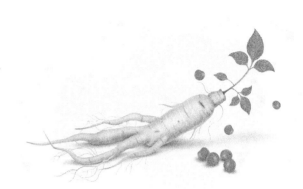

USES: *Ginseng is extensively utilized due to its adaptogenic properties, which assist the body in coping with stress and promote overall health. Additionally, it is used to improve physical performance, enhance cognitive function, and strengthen the immune system. Ginseng is frequently used in traditional medicine to treat a variety of diseases, including diabetes, hypertension, and erectile dysfunction.*

HABITATS: *Ginseng thrives in environments that are chilly and shady, such as mountainous forests. The plant requires rich, moist soil to develop, and it takes several years to mature. Ginseng is frequently grown in the United States, Canada, and China, where its medicinal properties are highly valued.*

ACTIVE PRINCIPLES: *Ginseng's therapeutic effects are due to a group of compounds called ginsenosides. It is believed that these compounds possess anti-inflammatory, antioxidant, and anti-cancer properties. In addition to polysaccharides, peptides, and fatty acids, ginseng also contains compounds that contribute to its health benefits.*

EFFECTS AND CONTRADICATIONS: *Ginseng is generally considered harmless for moderate consumption. However, ginseng in excessive doses can cause side effects such as headaches, insomnia, and digestive issues. Ginseng may interact with certain medications, including blood thinners and diabetes drugs, and expectant and breastfeeding women should avoid it.*

TRADITIONAL USES: *In traditional Chinese medicine, ginseng has been used for centuries to treat a variety of health conditions, including fatigue, tension, and sexual dysfunction. It is also used to improve physical and mental performance in traditional Korean medicine. Native Americans in the United States* used ginseng for its medicinal properties, and European settlers subsequently adopted it for its health benefits.

• *HAWTHORN*

USES: *Hawthorn is known for its cardiovascular benefits. It is used to support heart health, improve blood circulation, and regulate blood pressure. Hawthorn berries, leaves, and flowers are often used to make herbal preparations like tinctures, teas, and capsules.*

HABITATS: *Hawthorn is native to Europe, North America, and Asia. It grows in temperate climates and can be found in woodlands, hedges, and gardens.*

ACTIVE PRINCIPLES: *Hawthorn contains bioflavonoids, such as proanthocyanidins and quercetin, as well as cardiac glycosides and antioxidants.*

EFFECTS AND CONTRAINDICATIONS: *Hawthorn is generally considered safe when used as directed. However, it may interact with certain medications, including beta-blockers and nitrates. It is advisable to consult with a healthcare professional before using hawthorn, especially if you have a heart condition or are taking medication.*

TRADITIONAL USES: *Hawthorn has a long history of traditional use for heart-related conditions. It has been used to support heart function, strengthen the cardiovascular system, and reduce symptoms of heart failure.*

• *IVY*

USES: *Ivy is primarily used as an ornamental plant, but it also has some medicinal applications. Ivy extracts are used in traditional cough medicines and expectorants to help relieve coughs and promote respiratory health.*

HABITATS: *Ivy is native to Europe but can now be found in various regions around the world. It grows in forests, on walls, and as a climbing vine.*

ACTIVE PRINCIPLES: *Ivy contains saponins, including hederacoside C, as well as flavonoids and polyacetylenes.*

EFFECTS AND CONTRAINDICATIONS: *Ivy can cause skin irritation and allergic reactions in some individuals, especially when used topically. It should not be ingested or applied to open wounds.*

TRADITIONAL USES: *Ivy has been used traditionally to alleviate coughs, bronchitis, and respiratory congestion. It has also been used externally for its skin-soothing properties.*

• *JASMINE*

USES: *Jasmine is prized for its aromatic flowers and is commonly used in perfumes, teas, and essential oils. Jasmine tea is known for its calming properties and is often consumed for relaxation and stress relief.*

HABITATS: *Jasmine is native to tropical and subtropical regions and is widely cultivated for ornamental purposes. It thrives in warm climates and can be found in gardens and plantations.*

ACTIVE PRINCIPLES: *Jasmine flowers contain essential oils, including linalool and benzyl acetate, which contribute to its distinct fragrance and therapeutic properties. It also contains flavonoids and antioxidants.*

EFFECTS AND CONTRAINDICATIONS: *Jasmine is generally safe for most people when used in moderation. Its aroma and properties make it popular for relaxation and promoting a sense of well-being. However, some individuals may be sensitive to its fragrance. It is advisable to avoid excessive use or contact with jasmine oil, as it can cause skin irritation or allergic reactions in some people.*

TRADITIONAL USES: *Jasmine has a rich history of traditional uses in various cultures. It has been used for its calming and sedative effects, promoting relaxation, alleviating stress and anxiety, and enhancing mood. In traditional medicine, it has also been used to address digestive issues and stimulate appetite.*

• *KAVA*

USES: *Kava, also known as kava kava, is a plant traditionally used for its sedative and anxiolytic properties. It is consumed as a beverage made from the roots of the plant and is known for its relaxing effects.*

HABITATS: *Kava is native to the South Pacific islands and is cultivated in countries like Fiji, Vanuatu, and Samoa. It thrives in tropical environments and grows best in well-drained soil.*

ACTIVE PRINCIPLES: *Kava contains kavalactones, which are considered the primary active compounds responsible for its effects. The specific kavalactones present can vary depending on the variety and preparation method.*

EFFECTS AND CONTRAINDICATIONS: *Kava has a calming effect and is used to promote relaxation and reduce anxiety. However, it should be used with caution and under the guidance of a healthcare professional due to potential liver toxicity concerns. Long-term or excessive use of kava has been associated with rare cases of liver damage.*

TRADITIONAL USES: *Kava has a long history of traditional use in Pacific island cultures, where it is consumed in social and ceremonial settings to promote relaxation and enhance sociability. It has been used to alleviate symptoms of anxiety, stress, and insomnia.*

- **LAVENDER**

Lavender floral plant is a member of the mint family. Originating in the Mediterranean region, it is now grown and cultivated all over the globe. Lavender is an extensively utilized herb for its medicinal and aromatic qualities.

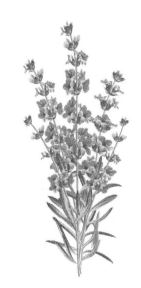

USES: *Lavender is utilized primarily for its soothing and sedative properties. It is frequently employed in aromatherapy to promote relaxation and alleviate tension and anxiety. In addition to calming and moisturizing the skin, lavender oil is also used to treat acne and other skin conditions. Additionally, it is utilized as a natural insect repellent and as a treatment for migraines and menstrual cramps.*

HABITATS: *Typically, lavender is cultivated in sunny, well-drained soils. It is commonly found in the Mediterranean region, but it is also cultivated in Europe, North America, and Australia, among other places. Lavender can be cultivated in both gardens and receptacles.*

ACTIVE PRINCIPLES: *Several active components in lavender are responsible for its therapeutic effects. These include terpenes-4-ol, linalool, and linalyl acetate. Due to the anti- inflammatory, analgesic, and anxiolytic properties of these compounds, lavender is an effective treatment for a variety of health conditions.*

EFFECTS AND CONTRAINDICATIONS: *Lavender is generally safe for use by the majority of individuals. However, lavender products may cause allergic reactions in some individuals. Additionally, ingestion of lavender oil can cause digestive issues such as vertigo and vomiting. Pregnant and nursing women should also avoid using lavender products, as there is insufficient data to ascertain their safety during pregnancy and breastfeeding.*

TRADITIONAL USES: *For centuries, lavender has been utilized for its medicinal properties. In traditional medicine, it is used to alleviate insomnia, anxiety, and depression, among other conditions. Lavender is also employed as a natural remedy for migraines and as a digestive aid. In aromatherapy, it is used to promote relaxation and reduce tension.*

• *LEMON BALM*

Lemon Balm is also known Melissa officinalis. This is an herb with a citrus scent that belongs to the mint family. It has been utilized for centuries due to its medicinal properties, and it is a popular herb used in infusions and aromatherapy. Here are some details about lemon balm, including its traditional uses, habitats, active ingredients, effects, and contraindications.

USES: *Due to its calming properties, lemon balm is frequently used as a natural remedy for anxiety and insomnia. Additionally, it is used to treat digestive issues like bloating, gas, and gastric cramps. Lemon balm has antiviral properties and is utilized to strengthen the immune system, particularly during cold and flu season. It has been used to treat cold sores and other skin conditions topically.*

HABITATS: *Lemon balm is native to Europe and the Mediterranean, but it can also be found in North America, Asia, and Australia, among other places. It thrives in well-drained, full-sun or moderate-shade soil. Lemon balm can reach a height of two feet and generate tiny white or yellow flowers.*

ACTIVE PRINCIPLES: *Lemon balm contains the active ingredients rosmarinic acid, citronellal, and eugenol. Rosmarinus acid is a potent antioxidant that defends the body against oxidative stress. Citronellal* is responsible for the citrus scent and anti-inflammatory properties of the plant. Cloves also contain eugenol, which has analgesic properties.

EFFECTS AND CONTRADICTIONS: *Lemon balm is generally regarded as harmless for moderate consumption. However, it may cause moderate nausea, dizziness, and abdominal pain as moderate side effects. Certain medications, including sedatives, thyroid medications, and blood thinners, can interact with lemon balm. Lemon balm can interfere with thyroid hormone secretion and should not be used by pregnant or breastfeeding women, as well as those with thyroid conditions.*

TRADITIONAL USES: *Lemon balm has been utilized for its medicinal properties for centuries. It was used to treat anxiety, insomnia, and digestive issues in ancient Greece and Rome. Additionally, it was utilized as a natural treatment for cold ulcers and other skin conditions. Lemon balm was used to cure liver and digestive disorders in traditional Chinese medicine.*

- *MINT*

Mint is an herbaceous plant that is native to Europe, Asia, and North America and is a member of the Lamiaceae family. It is utilized for its refreshing and energizing properties and is well-known for its intense aroma and flavor. There are numerous types of mint, such as peppermint, spearmint, and chocolate mint, each with a distinct flavor and fragrance.

USES: *Mint is commonly utilized for its medicinal and culinary benefits. It is frequently used to lend flavor to foods like salads, teas, and desserts. In aromatherapy, the oil extracted from mint leaves is used to promote relaxation and reduce tension. Additionally, mint is used to treat digestive issues such as nausea, bloating, and dyspepsia.*

HABITATS: *Growing in gardens, fields, and natural habitats such as meadows and forests, mint prefers moist soil and partial shade. Peppermint is cultivated in the United States, Europe, and Asia, whereas spearmint is cultivated more frequently in Europe.*

ACTIVE PRINCIPLES: *Several active compounds, including menthol, rosmarinic acid, and flavonoids, are present in mint. Menthol is responsible for the cooling and invigorating effect of mint, whereas rosmarinic acid has antioxidant properties that protect the body from free radical damage. Flavonoids are* anti-inflammatory plant compounds that may help reduce the risk of chronic diseases such as heart disease and cancer.

EFFECTS AND CONTRADICTIONS: *In moderate quantities, mint is generally considered safe for human consumption. Mint can cause adverse effects such as heartburn, headaches, and allergic reactions when consumed in excess. Mint oil should not be applied to the skin directly because it may cause irritation. Individuals with gastroesophageal reflux disease (GERD) should avoid consuming significant quantities of mint, as it may aggravate symptoms.*

TRADITIONAL USES: *Mint has been utilized for medicinal purposes for millennia. Mint was used to alleviate digestive issues and promote healthy digestion in ancient Greece and Rome. Mint is used in traditional Chinese medicine to treat migraines, fevers, and coughs. Native Americans utilized mint for pain relief and healing.*

- **NETTLE**

Nettle, also known as stinging nettle, is a perennial herbaceous plant that is widespread throughout the world's temperate regions. It has been employed in traditional medicine for centuries due to its numerous medicinal and nutritional properties.

USES: *Common uses for nettle include the treatment of allergies, joint inflammation, and urinary tract infections. Vitamin C, iron, and magnesium are among the many vitamins and minerals present in abundance. Additionally, nettle is used to treat respiratory conditions like asthma and hay fever. It is thought to possess anti-inflammatory, diuretic, and pain-relieving properties, making it a popular natural treatment for arthritis and other inflammatory conditions.*

HABITATS: *Nettle grows in a range of environments, including meadows, hedgerows, and disturbed areas. It prefers nutrient-rich soils and grows frequently near streams and other water sources. Nettle is a resilient plant that can withstand a wide range of temperatures and environmental conditions.*

ACTIVE PRINCIPLES: *Nettle contains an assortment of active compounds, such as flavonoids, carotenoids, and phenolic acids. Additionally, it is abundant in vitamins and minerals, including vitamins A, C, and K, iron, and magnesium. In addition to histamine, serotonin, and acetylcholine, the plant contains substances that contribute to its therapeutic properties.*

EFFECTS AND CONTRADICTIONS: *When consumed in moderation, stinging nettle is generally considered safe for most individuals. However, allergic reactions to nettle can cause skin irritation, itching, and edema in some individuals. Additionally, nettle can interact with certain medications, such as blood thinners and diuretics. Before using nettle as a treatment for any medical condition, it is crucial to consult a healthcare provider.*

TRADITIONAL USES: *Since ancient times, nettles have been utilized in traditional medicine. It has been utilized to treat a variety of conditions, such as arthritis, allergies, and urinary tract infections. Nettle is utilized in traditional Chinese medicine to strengthen the kidneys and cure asthma and other respiratory conditions. Nettle is used in Ayurvedic medicine to alleviate inflammation, rheumatism, and skin conditions.*

• OREGANO

Oregano is a perennial herb extensively used in traditional cooking and medicine. It is endemic to the Mediterranean and is a member of the mint family. Oregano's robust flavor and aroma make it a popular ingredient in a variety of cuisines, particularly Italian and Greek dishes.

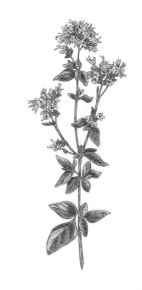

USES: *In addition to its culinary applications, oregano is used in traditional medicine due to its numerous health benefits. It is believed to have antibacterial, anti-inflammatory, and antioxidant properties. Oregano is employed for the treatment of respiratory infections, digestive issues, menstrual cramping, and urinary tract infections. It is also applied topically as a natural treatment for acne, eczema, and psoriasis.*

HABITATS: *Oregano is a resilient perennial that prefers well-drained soil and full sun. It can thrive in a range of environments, including rocky slopes, arid meadows, and scrublands. Originating in the*

Mediterranean region, oregano is now cultivated throughout the world, including in Europe, North America, and Asia.

ACTIVE PRINCIPLES: Carvacrol, thymol, rosmarinic acid, and flavonoids are some of the active ingredients found in oregano. These compounds account for the antimicrobial, antioxidant, and anti-inflammatory properties of the herb. Oregano contains the antimicrobial compounds carvacrol and thymol, which are particularly effective against bacteria and fungi.

EFFECTS AND CONTRADICTIONS: Oregano is generally harmless for human consumption and medicinal use. Nevertheless, it may induce allergic reactions in some people. As it may stimulate uterine contractions, it is also not recommended for expectant women. Undiluted oregano oil should not be applied topically, as it may cause skin irritation.

TRADITIONAL USES: Oregano has a lengthy history of medicinal applications. The ancient Greeks and Romans used it to treat digestive disorders, respiratory infections, and skin conditions, among others. Oregano is used in traditional Chinese medicine to alleviate fever, vomiting, and diarrhea. In Ayurvedic medicine, it is also used to promote digestion and treat respiratory and digestive disorders.

• PEPPERMINT

Peppermint (Mentha x piperita) is a hybrid plant of water mint and spearmint with a distinct aroma and revitalizing flavor. Native to Europe and Asia, peppermint is now cultivated worldwide for its numerous purposes and benefits.

USES: For its fresh and minty flavor, peppermint is frequently used in cooking and baking. Additionally, it is utilized in the production of toothpaste, mouthwash, and detergents. Peppermint oil is used in aromatherapy to alleviate tension and anxiety and in topical treatments for its calming and cooling properties. Due to its digestive properties, peppermint tea is ingested to alleviate symptoms of bloating, gas, and indigestion.

HABITATS: Peppermint prefers cool, moist conditions and is typically located in shady areas near streams and lakes. It is a perennial plant that can reach a height of three feet and produces purple blossoms in the summer.

ACTIVE PRINCIPLES: *There are several active compounds in peppermint, including menthol, menthone, and eucalyptol. These compounds are responsible for the aroma and flavor of peppermint as well as its medicinal properties. Menthol's cooling and analgesic properties make it a popular constituent in topical pain-relieving products.*

EFFECTS AND CONTRADICTIONS: *In moderation, peppermint is generally considered safe. However, excessive consumption of peppermint tea or oil may result in adverse effects such as heartburn, nausea, and allergic reactions. As it can cause irritation, vertigo, and even convulsions in some people, peppermint oil should not be applied directly to the skin or ingested in large quantities. Individuals with gastroesophageal reflux disease (GERD) or gastrointestinal issues should also avoid peppermint, as it can exacerbate these conditions.*

TRADITIONAL USES: *For centuries, peppermint has been utilized for its medicinal properties. It was utilized in ancient Egypt, Greece, and Rome for its digestive properties and in traditional Chinese and Ayurvedic medicine to treat a variety of maladies, including headaches, nausea, and respiratory issues. In Europe, peppermint was frequently used to alleviate menstrual cramping and facilitate childbirth. Peppermint is still utilized for its therapeutic properties and is a common component in many natural remedies and dietary supplements.*

- **QUINOA**

USES: *Quinoa is a nutritious grain that is often used as a staple food due to its high protein content and essential amino acids. It can be cooked and used in various dishes such as salads, soups, and as a substitute for rice.*

HABITATS: *Quinoa is native to the Andean region of South America, particularly Peru, Bolivia, and Ecuador. It grows best in high-altitude areas with cool temperatures and well- drained soils.*

ACTIVE PRINCIPLES: *Quinoa is rich in protein, dietary fiber, vitamins (such as B vitamins and vitamin E), minerals (including iron, magnesium, and phosphorus), and antioxidants.*

EFFECTS AND CONTRAINDICATIONS: *Quinoa is generally safe for consumption and is well-tolerated by most individuals. However, some people may experience digestive issues or allergic reactions* to quinoa. It is advisable to rinse quinoa thoroughly before cooking to remove saponins, which can cause a bitter taste.

TRADITIONAL USES: Quinoa has been cultivated and consumed by indigenous peoples in the Andean region for thousands of years. It was a vital part of their diet and played a significant role in their traditional rituals and ceremonies.

• ROSEMARY

Rosemary is a perennial herb native to the Mediterranean region (Rosmarinus officinalis). It is a member of the mint family, and its culinary and medicinal applications are well known. Here are some specific details about the plant:

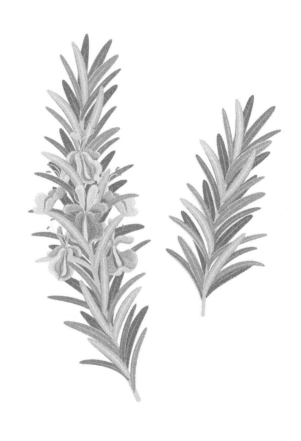

USES: Rosemary is a prevalent culinary herb used to add flavor to a variety of foods, including soups, stews, meats, and bread. It has a strong, pungent aroma and a flavor that is mildly bitter. Due to its pleasant fragrance, the herb is also utilized in the production of perfumes, cosmetics, and soaps. Rosemary is well-known for its medicinal properties in addition to its culinary applications. It has been used historically to treat a variety of conditions, including headaches, indigestion, and muscle discomfort. In aromatherapy, rosemary oil is commonly used to reduce tension and anxiety and enhance concentration.

HABITATS: Rosemary is a hardy plant that thrives in warm, arid, and rocky soil. It can also be cultivated in California, Australia, and South Africa, which have climates similar to the Mediterranean.

ACTIVE PRINCIPLES: *Rosemary contains a variety of active ingredients, including rosmarinic acid, carnosic acid, and caffeic acid. These compounds account for the antioxidant and anti-inflammatory properties of the herb. Rosemary also contains essential oils, including cineole and camphor, which contribute to the plant's distinctive aroma.*

EFFECTS AND CONTRADICTIONS: *Consuming rosemary in moderate quantities as a food or supplement is generally safe. Nevertheless, it may induce allergic reactions in some people. In large doses, rosemary oil can induce vomiting, spasms, and convulsions. Women who are pregnant or nursing should avoid using rosemary oil because it may induce uterine contractions. Additionally, individuals with epilepsy or hypertension should consult a physician prior to taking rosemary supplements, as it may interact with certain medications.*

TRADITIONAL USES: *Rosemary has been used in traditional medicine to cure a variety of ailments for centuries. In ancient Greece, rosemary was used to stimulate hair growth and enhance memory. The herb was utilized in traditional Chinese medicine to treat digestive disorders and menstrual cramping. During the Middle Ages, rosemary was also used to ward off evil entities and protect against the plague.*

- ***SAGE***

Sage is a perennial herb that is extensively used in traditional medicine and in cooking. It is indigenous to the Mediterranean region but is now widespread, including in North America and Asia. Sage's uses, habitats, active principles, effects, and traditional applications are described below.

USES: *Sage has been utilized in traditional medicine for centuries. It has antimicrobial, anti-inflammatory, and antioxidant properties. Sage has been used to treat numerous afflictions, including digestive problems, sore throats, respiratory infections, and menopausal symptoms. It is also commonly used to impart flavor to dishes, especially in Mediterranean cuisine.*

HABITATS: *Sage flourishes in mild, arid climates and grows in rocky, well-drained soil. It is endemic to the Mediterranean region as well as portions of North America, Asia, and Europe. Sage is commonly cultivated as an ornamental plant in gardens and is easy to cultivate in containers.*

ACTIVE PRINCIPLES: *Sage contains numerous active ingredients, including essential oils, flavonoids, and phenolic acids. Sage's essential oil contains compounds that contribute to its medicinal properties,* *including thujone, camphor, and cineole. Flavonoids and phenolic acids are potent antioxidants that assist in protecting the body from oxidative stress.*

EFFECTS AND CONTRADICTIONS: *Sage has many potential health benefits, but it is crucial to note that improper use can have negative effects. Sage is toxic in large doses and may cause vertigo, convulsions, and other neurological symptoms. Sage is not advised for expectant women because it may stimulate the uterus and induce contractions. Individuals with a history of seizures and those taking medications for high blood pressure should also use it with caution.*

TRADITIONAL USES: *Sage has been utilized in traditional medicine for millennia. It was used for its medicinal properties by the ancient Greeks and Romans, as well as by indigenous cultures from all over the globe. Sage has been used to treat a variety of maladies, including digestive issues, sore throat, respiratory infections, and menopausal symptoms, in traditional medicine. Native American cultures use it frequently in smudging ceremonies to purify the air and promote spiritual healing.*

• THE ST. JOHN'S WORT

St. John's Wort, also known as Hypericum perforatum, is a medicinal plant that has been used for centuries. It is a perennial plant native to Europe that is also found in Asia, Africa, and North America. Here are some details about its traditional uses, habitats, active ingredients, effects, and contraindications:

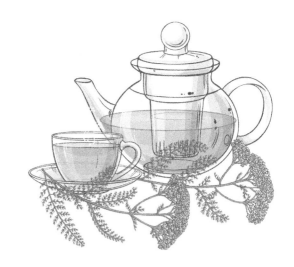

USES: *St. John's Wort has been used to treat depression, anxiety, sleep disorders, and nerve discomfort, among other conditions. Serotonin, dopamine, and norepinephrine, which are involved in mood regulation, are believed to be responsible for its effectiveness. St. John's Wort is therefore frequently used as a natural alternative to antidepressants.*

HABITATS: *St. John's Wort is a resilient plant that can thrive in a variety of environments, including meadows, fields, and woodland borders. It requires full sun and well-drained loam to flourish.*

ACTIVE PRINCIPLES: *St. John's Wort contains the active ingredients hypericin, hyperforin, and flavonoids. It is believed that hypericin and hyperforin are responsible for the antidepressant effects of St. John's Wort, while flavonoids have anti-inflammatory and antioxidant properties.*

EFFECTS AND CONTRADICTIONS: *The effectiveness of St. John's Wort in treating mild to moderate depression has been demonstrated. It may interact, however, with antidepressants, birth control drugs, and blood thinners. Therefore, it is essential to consult a healthcare professional prior to consuming St. John's Wort if you are currently taking medication. It can also cause photosensitivity, so excessive sun exposure should be avoided while taking St. John's Wort.*

TRADITIONAL USES: *St. John's Wort has been used for centuries in traditional medicine. It was used to treat a variety of ailments, including incisions and inflammation, in ancient Greece. It was used in traditional Chinese medicine to alleviate depression, anxiety, and digestive disorders. It was used to treat nervous disorders and alleviate discomfort in medieval Europe. St. John's Wort is still extensively used for its medicinal properties and is a common ingredient in dietary supplements.*

- **THYME**

USES: *Thyme is a culinary herb with a distinct aromatic flavor and is commonly used to season a variety of dishes, including soups, stews, meats, and vegetables. It is also used in herbal teas and as an ingredient in natural remedies.*

HABITATS: *Thyme is native to the Mediterranean region but is now widely cultivated in various parts of the world. It prefers well-drained soil, plenty of sunlight, and a warm climate.*

ACTIVE PRINCIPLES: *Thyme contains essential oils, including thymol, which possesses antimicrobial*

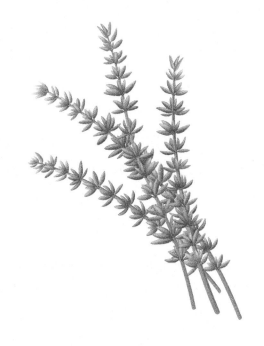

properties. It also contains flavonoids, phenolic compounds, and vitamins.

EFFECTS AND CONTRAINDICATIONS: *Thyme is generally safe when used in moderation as a culinary herb. However, concentrated thyme oil or high doses of thyme may cause irritation or allergic reactions. Pregnant women should avoid consuming large amounts of thyme.*

TRADITIONAL USES: *Thyme has been used in traditional medicine for its expectorant and antiseptic properties. It has been employed to relieve respiratory conditions, coughs, and sore throats. Additionally, it has been used topically as a natural antiseptic for wounds and skin infections.*

• *TURMERIC*

Turmeric is scientifically known as Curcuma. Turmeric is a perennial herbaceous plant pertaining to the Zingiberaceae family. It is indigenous to South Asia and has been used in Ayurvedic medicine for centuries to address a variety of ailments. Curcumin, the active ingredient in turmeric, is responsible for the spice's vibrant yellow hue.

USES: *In Indian and Middle Eastern cuisine, turmeric is commonly used as a spice to give flavor and color to dishes such as curry. In addition to its culinary applications, turmeric has medicinal properties. It has been used to treat a variety of conditions, including arthritis, digestive issues, and skin problems, due to its anti-inflammatory, antioxidant, and antimicrobial properties.*

HABITATS: *In tropical and subtropical regions, turmeric is cultivated extensively, particularly in India. It thrives in well-drained, high-temperature soil and requires abundant rainfall. Up to three feet in height, turmeric plants have large, green leaves and yellow or white blossoms.*

ACTIVE PRINCIPLES: *Curcumin, the active constituent in turmeric, has been demonstrated to have potent anti-inflammatory and antioxidant properties. Curcumin is a polyphenol responsible for the vibrant yellow color of turmeric. Additionally, turmeric contains essential oils, turmerones, and curcuminoids.*

EFFECTS AND CONTRADICTIONS: *As a spice or dietary supplement, turmeric is generally considered safe when consumed in moderate quantities. However, some individuals may experience adverse effects, including stomach distress, nausea, and diarrhea. Turmeric may interact with certain medications, such as blood thinners, and should be used cautiously in these instances.*

TRADITIONAL USES: *The use of turmeric in Ayurvedic and traditional Chinese medicine dates back centuries. It has been used to treat numerous conditions, including digestive issues, skin issues, and joint discomfort. Turmeric is used as a natural remedy for coughs, colds, and other respiratory conditions in Ayurvedic medicine. Additionally, it is used to improve digestion, strengthen the immune system, and promote healthy skin. Turmeric is used in traditional Chinese medicine to treat menstrual pain, liver and gallbladder issues, and to promote healthy blood circulation.*

• *UVA URSI (BEARBERRY)*

USES: *Uva Ursi is an herb traditionally used to treat urinary tract infections, kidney stones, and bladder issues. It is known for its diuretic and antiseptic properties.*

HABITATS: *Uva Ursi is native to North America, Europe, and Asia, and it typically grows in mountainous regions with acidic, well-drained soils.*

ACTIVE PRINCIPLES: *Uva Ursi contains hydroquinone glycosides, such as arbutin, which has antimicrobial properties. It also contains tannins, flavonoids, and volatile oils.*

EFFECTS AND CONTRAINDICATIONS: *Uva Ursi should be used under the guidance of a healthcare professional, as it may interact with certain medications and may not be suitable for everyone. Prolonged or excessive use can lead to side effects such as digestive upset or liver damage.*

TRADITIONAL USES: *Uva Ursi has a long history of traditional use by Native American tribes and European herbalists. It has been used as a urinary antiseptic and astringent, believed to help alleviate urinary tract infections and promote kidney health.*

- **VALERIAN**

USES: *Valerian is an herb commonly used as a natural remedy to promote relaxation, relieve anxiety, and improve sleep quality. It is available in various forms, including capsules, tinctures, and teas.*

HABITATS: *Valerian is native to Europe and parts of Asia but is now cultivated worldwide. It prefers moist soil and is often found growing near streams, rivers, and damp meadows.*

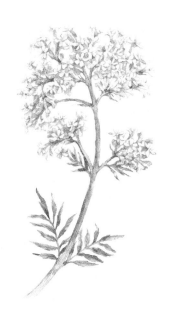

ACTIVE PRINCIPLES: *Valerian root contains several active compounds, including valerenic acid and valerenol, which are believed to have sedative and anxiolytic effects. It also contains volatile oils and alkaloids.*

EFFECTS AND CONTRAINDICATIONS: *Valerian is generally considered safe for short-term use. However, it may cause drowsiness, dizziness, or an upset stomach in some individuals. It is not recommended for pregnant or breastfeeding women, and it may interact with certain medications.*

TRADITIONAL USES: *Valerian has a long history of use in traditional medicine as a calming and sleep-promoting herb. It was commonly employed to alleviate nervousness, restlessness, and sleep disturbances.*

- **WHEATGRASS**

USES: *Wheatgrass refers to the young shoots of the wheat plant, Triticum aestivum. It is consumed as a dietary supplement in the form of fresh juice, powder, or capsules. Wheatgrass is believed to have various health benefits due to its high content of vitamins, minerals, chlorophyll, and antioxidants.*

HABITATS: *Wheatgrass is cultivated in many parts of the world, both indoors (hydroponically) and outdoors, under controlled conditions. It requires well-drained soil, adequate sunlight, and regular watering.*

ACTIVE PRINCIPLES: *Wheatgrass is rich in vitamins (such as vitamins A, C, and E), minerals (including iron, calcium, and magnesium), enzymes, and chlorophyll.*

EFFECTS AND CONTRAINDICATIONS: *Wheatgrass is generally safe for most individuals. However, some people may experience nausea, stomach upset, or allergic reactions. It is advisable to start with small amounts and monitor your body's response.*

TRADITIONAL USES: *Wheatgrass has been used for centuries in traditional medicine, particularly in Ayurveda, as a rejuvenating tonic and for its detoxifying properties. It is believed to support overall health, boost immunity, and enhance vitality.*

• *XANTHAN GUM (DERIVED FROM PLANTS)*

USES: *Xanthan gum is a polysaccharide derived from plants, primarily corn, wheat, or soy. It is commonly used as a thickening agent, stabilizer, or emulsifier in various food products, including sauces, dressings, and gluten-free baking.*

HABITATS: *Xanthan gum is not derived from a specific plant but is produced through the fermentation of sugars using the Xanthomonas campestris bacterium. The bacteria are cultivated in a laboratory setting.*

ACTIVE PRINCIPLES: *Xanthan gum is composed of long chains of glucose molecules. It forms a gel-like substance when combined with water, providing viscosity and stability to food products.*

EFFECTS AND CONTRAINDICATIONS: *Xanthan gum is generally considered safe for consumption. However, some individuals may experience digestive discomfort or allergic reactions. It is commonly used in gluten-free products as a substitute for gluten, making them more accessible to individuals with gluten intolerance or celiac disease.*

TRADITIONAL USES: *Xanthan gum is a relatively modern food ingredient and does not have a traditional history of use as an herb or plant.*

• *YARROW*

Yarrow, also known as Achillea millefolium, is a flowering plant that is indigenous to Europe and Asia but can now be found worldwide. It has a lengthy history of use in traditional medicine, and its active components have been the subject of extensive research regarding their potential health benefits.

31

USES: *Yarrow has been used for a variety of medicinal purposes, such as aiding digestion, reducing fever, and treating ulcers. Additionally, it is frequently used as a diuretic and to relieve menstrual cramping. Yarrow has also been applied topically as a poultice or salve to promote wound healing and decrease inflammation.*

HABITATS: *Yarrow grows in a diversity of habitats, including meadows, grasslands, and roadside margins. It is a resilient plant that thrives in deficient soil conditions and is frequently used in landscaping and gardening.*

ACTIVE CONCEPTS: *Yarrow contains volatile oils, flavonoids, and tannins as its active ingredients. Yarrow flavonoids, including apigenin and luteolin, have anti-inflammatory and antioxidant properties. Tannins are a form of polyphenol with anti-inflammatory and astringent properties. It is believed that the volatile oils in yarrow, including chamazulene and cineole, have anti-inflammatory and antimicrobial properties.*

EFFECTS AND CONTRADICTIONS: *When taken as directed, yarrow is generally regarded as safe. You should be aware of a few possible adverse effects and contraindications, though. Some people, particularly those who are allergic to members of the Asteraceae family of plants, including ragweed and chrysanthemums, may experience allergic reactions when exposed to yarrow. It may also interact with other drugs, such as blood thinners and diabetes medications. Avoid using yarrow during pregnancy and breastfeeding, as it may stimulate the uterus and impact milk production.*

TRADITIONAL USES: *The use of yarrow in traditional medicine dates back to ancient Greece and Rome. The ancient Greeks employed yarrow as a natural medicine for menstruation- related symptoms as well as for wounds, fever, and digestive problems. Yarrow is utilized in traditional Chinese medicine to improve circulation and mitigate pain. Native American cultures employed yarrow for a range of medical conditions, such as respiratory problems and fever reduction.*

• ZEDOARY

USES: *Zedoary is a rhizome of a tropical plant (Curcuma zedoaria) and is used as a culinary spice and herbal remedy. It is known for its digestive properties and is often used in traditional medicine to promote healthy digestion.*

HABITATS: *Zedoary is native to India and Southeast Asia. It thrives in tropical climates and is cultivated for its rhizomes, which are harvested for various purposes.*

ACTIVE PRINCIPLES: *Zedoary contains essential oils, curcuminoids (including curcumin), and other bioactive compounds. It shares some similarities with turmeric, another member of the ginger family.*

EFFECTS AND CONTRAINDICATIONS: *Zedoary is generally safe when consumed in culinary amounts. However, concentrated zedoary extracts or high doses may cause stomach upset or interact with certain medications. Pregnant women should avoid excessive consumption.*

TRADITIONAL USES: *Zedoary has been used in traditional Ayurvedic and Chinese medicine for its digestive and anti-inflammatory properties. It is often used to relieve indigestion, bloating, and stomach discomfort. It is also used externally as a poultice for wounds or skin conditions.*

• ZINC

Zinc is a crucial mineral needed for a number of body processes, including DNA synthesis, wound healing, and immune system health. Various foods, such as meat, shellfish, and legumes, naturally contain it. In a nutritional supplement, zinc is additionally offered in pills, capsules, and lozenges.

USES: *Numerous uses for zinc exist, including the treatment of zinc deficiency, immune system support, and wound healing. Additionally, it is used to treat diarrhea, colds, and acne. The potential of zinc to shorten the length and intensity of cold symptoms, as well as its possible anti- inflammatory effects, have both been explored.*

HABITATS: *Several foods, including red meat, poultry, shellfish, beans, nuts, and whole grains, contain zinc. There are also zinc supplements available, and you can get them online and at most health food stores.*

ACTIVE CONCEPTS: *Zinc is a crucial mineral needed for numerous biological processes. It contributes to the synthesis of proteins, DNA and RNA synthesis, and cell division. Additionally, zinc aids in wound healing and immune system function. Zinc gluconate, zinc acetate, zinc citrate, or zinc oxide are all possible ingredients in zinc supplements.*

EFFECTS AND CONTRADICTIONS: *When taken in large doses, zinc supplements can have unwanted side effects such as diarrhea, vomiting, and nausea. The use of high-dose zinc supplements* over a long period of time may also raise the risk of prostate cancer. Additionally, certain drugs, such as antibiotics, diuretics, and blood pressure medications, might interact negatively with zinc supplementation. Zinc supplements should not be taken by those with specific medical disorders, such as hemochromatosis and Wilson's disease.

TRADITIONAL USES: Since ancient times, people have employed zinc for its therapeutic benefits. Zinc has been used in traditional Chinese medicine to cure a number of ailments, such as fever, diarrhea, and sore throats. Zinc is utilized in Ayurvedic medicine to support a healthy digestive system, lower inflammation, and enhance immune system performance. Zinc is a mineral that is used in Western herbal medicine to treat acne, speed up the healing of wounds, and strengthen the immune system.

Chapter 2

DRYING PROCESSES

By exposing a substance to heat, air, or a mixture of the two, it is dried, which removes any remaining moisture. Foods including fruits, vegetables, and meats, as well as herbs, spices, and other plant components, can all be preserved by drying. A material's weight and volume can be reduced through drying, which makes it simpler to carry and store. There are various drying techniques, each with benefits and drawbacks: The oldest and most convenient way of drying is in the sun. It entails leaving the material out in the open, exposed to air and sunlight until it has fully dried. Sun drying is cheap and doesn't call for any specific tools. However, depending on the weather, it can take many days to finish.

- **Drying by Air:** To dry by air, you must hang the cloth in a place with good ventilation so that the air may circulate around it. For herbs, spices, and flowers, this procedure is frequently employed. Although it is a quick and inexpensive approach, air drying might take several days and is subject to the weather.

- **Drying in an oven:** Drying in an oven entail putting the material in and heating it for a long time at a low temperature. Fruits, vegetables, and meats are frequently prepared using this approach. Compared to sun and air drying, oven drying is quicker and gives you more control over the drying temperature. However, it can be pricey and calls for a special oven.

- **Drying with a Dehydrator:** A dehydrator is a specialized tool used to dry food and other materials. Heat and air are combined in dehydrators to remove moisture from the material. Dehydrators offer more temperature and humidity control than other drying techniques and are faster. They can, however, be pricey and run on electricity.

- **Drying by freeze:** Drying by freeze entails freezing the material and then removing the moisture with a vacuum. Foods such as fruits, vegetables, and meats, as well as medicines and other medical supplies, are frequently preserved using this technique. The most expensive drying technique, freeze drying, also retains most of the material's nutritional value.

COLD DRYING

Cold drying, commonly referred to as freeze-drying or lyophilization, is a heat-free method of eliminating moisture from products. The quality and integrity of many things, including food, medications, and biological materials, are frequently preserved using this method.

The product is frozen at extremely low temperatures, usually between -40°C and -80°C, as part of the cold drying process. The product is frozen, and then a vacuum is used to sublimate (directly turn ice into vapor without melting) the moisture out of the product. A dry, powdered product is the result of this procedure, which may be kept for longer periods of time without losing quality or nutritional content. The nutritional value and flavor of the product are two of the key benefits of cold drying. Cold drying does not subject the food to high temperatures or airflow, unlike other drying techniques like hot air drying or spray drying, which can harm the product's nutrition and flavor. The quality of delicate products, such as fruits, vegetables, and herbs, can thus be preserved.

The ability to prolong a product's shelf life is another benefit of cold drying. Cold drying prevents the development of germs and mold, which can ruin a product and shorten its shelf life, by removing moisture. This makes it a well-liked technique for preserving medicines, biological products, and other delicate goods that need a lengthy shelf life. Compared to other drying techniques, cold drying is also more eco-friendly. In contrast to hot air drying, which consumes a lot of energy to heat the air, cold drying utilizes less energy and doesn't create any waste or harmful pollutants. As a result, it is a more environmentally friendly form of drying that can lessen the negative effects of manufacturing and production procedures.

In contrast to other drying techniques like hot air drying or spray drying, cold drying is more expensive. This is due to the fact that it necessitates specialized equipment and a prolonged drying period, both of which might raise the production cost. Additionally, because the procedure is more labor-intensive, trained experts are needed to monitor it and guarantee the quality of the finished product.

HOT DRYING

High temperatures are used during the hot drying process to dry food goods. By heating the food product to a high temperature, usually above 60 °C (140 °F), the process evaporates the meal's moisture content. The process of hot drying is frequently used to produce dried fruits, vegetables, and meats.

There are various processes involved in the hot drying process. The food item is first cleaned and ready for drying. The food is then put into a drying chamber, which is usually heated with gas or electricity, to finish drying. The food is surrounded by hot air, which causes the moisture to evaporate and produce a dried product. Compared to other drying techniques, hot drying has a number of benefits. Because the moisture content is quickly evaporated by the high temperatures, it is a quick and effective way to dry food products. Due to the fact that high temperatures do not affect the food's nutrient content, this process also aids in maintaining the food's nutritional value.

Hot drying, however, also has certain drawbacks. As a result of the high temperatures utilized in this process, the meal may lose some of its flavor and texture and become less appetizing. As the drying chamber must be heated to a high temperature, hot drying can also be energy-intensive.

In general, hot drying is a popular technique for food product drying, especially for producing dried fruits, vegetables, and meats. While it has many benefits, including being rapid and effective, it also has some drawbacks, like changing the flavor and texture of the food. Hot drying must be done carefully and in line with food safety laws, just like any other technique of food processing.

WHAT A DRYER IS

A dryer is a device that removes water or moisture from a variety of objects, including clothing, textiles, and food items. In order to remove moisture from the material and leave it dry, the dryer uses a combination of heat and airflow.

Dryers come in a variety of designs, each intended for a particular application. For instance, a clothes dryer is made primarily for drying clothes, and it normally dries the fabric using warm air. In order to remove moisture from food goods, such as fruits and vegetables, a food dryer may employ a combination of heat and airflow or low temperatures and a vacuum.

Dryers exist in a variety of sizes and capacities, in addition to the specialized purposes for which they are designed. Smaller dryers, such as those found in homes to dry clothes, are usually made to handle smaller loads. Larger dryers, such as those seen in industrial settings, are built to process much higher material quantities and may even be made to run continuously for long periods of time.

Typically, using a dryer requires inserting the item and selecting the proper drying cycle. The moisture in the textile will subsequently be removed by the dryer using a mix of heat and airflow. The kind and quantity of the material being dried, together with the dryer's particular settings, will all affect how long the drying cycle lasts. A dryer is a device that uses heat and airflow to remove moisture from a variety of materials. Dryers are available in a wide variety of sizes and capacities, each with a different type that is intended for a particular application. A dryer's normal function entails inserting the material, selecting the correct drying cycle, and waiting for the dryer to remove the moisture.

COLLECTION AND STORAGE

A large number of businesses, such as agriculture, food manufacturing, and pharmaceuticals, place a high value on collection and storage. To ensure that the materials or goods are of high quality and free of contaminants, a meticulous collection of the materials or products must be made. Equally crucial is storage, which maintains the items' or materials' quality over time.

It is crucial to have a clear grasp of the desired qualities and properties before gathering materials or items. For instance, crops are often harvested in agriculture at a specified time to guarantee that they are at the ideal stage of growth. Similar to this, raw ingredients are gathered for food manufacturing based on their quality and freshness.

Once materials or goods have been gathered, it's critical to appropriately store them to preserve their quality. Degradation, contamination, and spoilage can all be avoided with proper storage. Depending on the material or product, particular storage needs may include elements like temperature, humidity, and light exposure.

Specialized equipment may be utilized for collection and storage in a variety of sectors. Materials may be gathered and stored, for instance, in clean rooms or specialized refrigeration units in the pharmaceutical sector. Crops may be harvested in agriculture using specialized equipment and then stored in silos or other storage facilities.

In conclusion, collecting and storage are vital components of many businesses and are essential to preserving the integrity and security of raw materials and finished goods. Utilizing the right strategies for collection and storage can help protect materials and products from degradation, contamination, and spoilage while also ensuring their high quality.

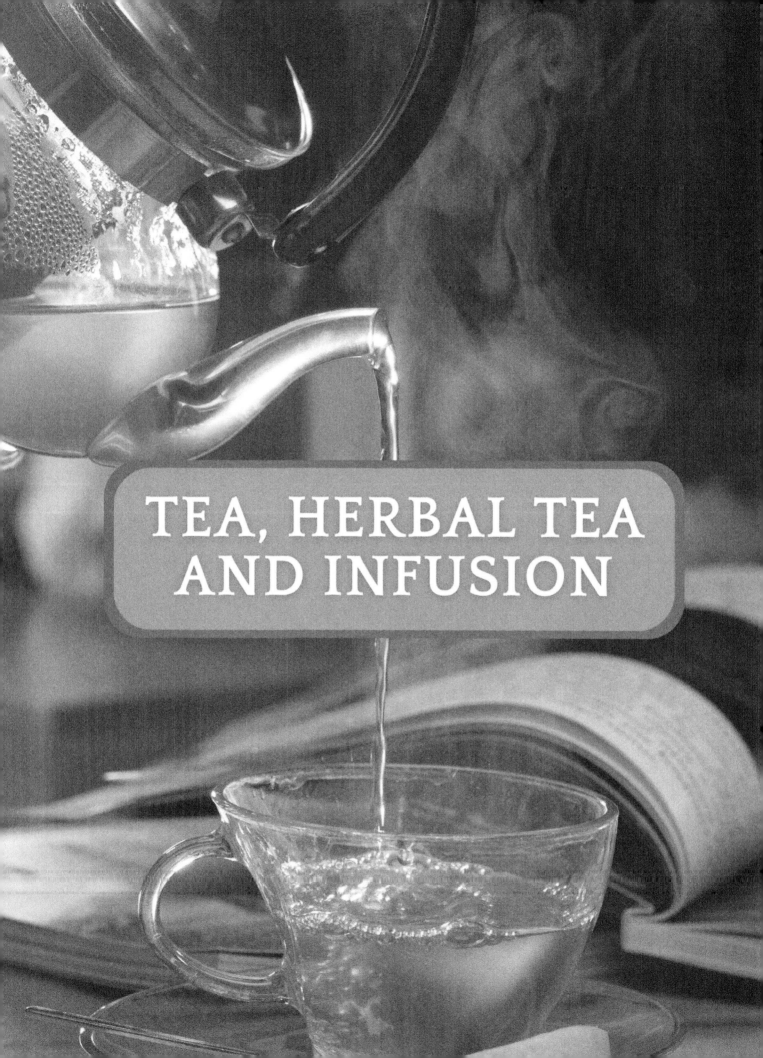

TEA, HERBAL TEA AND INFUSION

Chapter 1

INTRODUCTION TO TEA, HERBAL TEA, AND INFUSION

Tea, herbal tea, and infusion are three distinct types of beverages that are often consumed for their therapeutic benefits, flavor, and aroma. Although these terms are sometimes used interchangeably, they are actually quite different from one another in terms of their ingredients, preparation methods, and nutritional properties. Here is a breakdown of each:

- **Tea:**

Tea is a beverage made by steeping the leaves of the Camellia sinensis plant in hot water. The most common types of tea are black tea, green tea, oolong tea, and white tea, all of which come from the same plant, but are processed differently. Black tea is fully oxidized, green tea is not oxidized, oolong tea is partially oxidized, and white tea is made from the youngest and most tender tea leaves. Tea contains caffeine, antioxidants, and other nutrients that have been shown to improve brain function, reduce the risk of chronic diseases, and enhance mood and well-being.

- **Herbal Tea:**

Herbal tea, also known as tisane, is a beverage made from steeping the leaves, flowers, stems, and roots of various plants and herbs in hot water. Unlike tea, herbal tea does not contain any leaves from the Camellia sinensis plant. Some of the most popular herbal teas include chamomile, peppermint, ginger, rooibos, and hibiscus. Herbal tea has been used for centuries as a natural remedy for various ailments such as insomnia, anxiety, digestive issues, and menstrual cramps. Herbal teas are caffeine-free and contain a variety of beneficial plant compounds that may have anti-inflammatory, antibacterial, and antioxidant properties.

- **Infusion:**

Infusion refers to a method of preparing tea or herbal tea by steeping the ingredients in hot water for an extended period of time, usually 5-10 minutes. This allows the water to absorb the flavor and nutrients of the plant material. Infusions can be made with a wide variety of ingredients, including tea leaves, herbs, fruits, and spices. Some popular infusions include chai tea, fruit tea, and iced tea.

In summary, tea, herbal tea, and infusion are all delicious and healthy beverages that offer unique benefits. Tea comes from the Camellia sinensis plant and contains caffeine and antioxidants. Herbal tea is made from various plants and herbs and is caffeine-free. J8

DIFFERENCE BETWEEN TEA, HERBAL TEA AND INFUSION

Tea, herbal, and infusion are all popular hot beverages, but they differ in their ingredients and preparation methods.

- **Tea:**

Tea is made from the leaves of the Camellia sinensis plant. The leaves are harvested, withered, rolled, and dried to create various types of tea, including black, green, oolong, and white tea. The taste, aroma, and color of tea vary depending on factors such as the type of tea plant, the location where it is grown, and the processing method used.

- **Herbal tea:**

Herbal tea is made by steeping various parts of plants such as leaves, flowers, seeds, roots, and bark in hot water. Examples of herbs commonly used to make herbal tea include chamomile, peppermint, ginger, and rooibos. Unlike tea made from the tea plant, herbal tea does not contain caffeine and has a milder flavor.

- **Infusion:**

Infusion is a beverage made by steeping a combination of ingredients, including herbs, fruits, flowers, spices, and even tea leaves, in hot water. Infusions are typically made with a higher proportion of ingredients than tea or herbal tea and may be steeped for longer periods to extract maximum flavor. Infusions can be made with a single ingredient or a combination of several, and can be enjoyed hot or cold.

In summary, tea is made from the Camellia sinensis plant, herbal tea is made from steeping various parts of plants, and infusions are made by steeping a combination of ingredients in hot water. Each has its own unique flavor, aroma, and health benefits, making them popular choices for different occasions and preferences.

FEATURES OF TEA, HERBAL TEA AND INFUSION

Tea:

- Caffeine content: Tea is a natural source of caffeine, and the amount of caffeine varies depending on the type of tea. Black tea tends to have the highest caffeine content, followed by oolong, green, and white tea.

- Antioxidants: Tea contains antioxidants known as polyphenols, which can help protect against cellular damage and may have numerous health benefits.

- Varieties: Tea comes in many different varieties and flavors, including black tea, green tea, white tea, oolong tea, and others.

- Preparation: To make tea, tea leaves are steeped in hot water for several minutes, and the resulting beverage can be enjoyed hot or iced.

- Cultural significance: Tea has played an important role in many cultures throughout history, and it remains a popular beverage today.

Herbal Tea:

- Caffeine-free: Most herbal teas are naturally caffeine-free, making them a good choice for those who want to avoid caffeine.

- Flavor variety: Herbal tea comes in many different flavors, depending on the herbs, flowers, or fruits used in the blend.

- Health benefits: Depending on the herbs used, herbal tea can provide various health benefits, such as reducing inflammation, aiding digestion, or promoting relaxation.

- Preparation: Herbal tea is typically prepared by steeping herbs, flowers, or fruits in hot water for several minutes.

- Relaxation: Many herbal teas are known for their calming properties and can be enjoyed as a relaxing beverage before bedtime.

Infusion:

- Versatility: Infusions can be made from a wide range of plant materials, including dried fruits, herbs, spices, and flowers.

- Flavor variety: Like herbal tea, infusion offers a wide range of flavors and can be customized based on personal preferences.

- Caffeine content: Infusions made from some plant materials, such as yerba mate or guayusa, may contain caffeine, while others are naturally caffeine-free.

- Preparation: Infusions are typically prepared by steeping plant materials in hot water for several minutes.

- Health benefits: Depending on the plant materials used, infusions may offer various health benefits, such as providing vitamins and minerals, supporting digestion, or boosting the immune system.

CORRECT USE OF INGREDIENTS

Tea, herbal tea, and infusions are all popular beverages that can offer numerous health benefits. One of the most important aspects of making a great cup of any of these drinks is using the correct ingredients.

When making tea, the type of tea leaves used will determine the flavor and health benefits of the drink. For example, green tea leaves are known for their antioxidant properties, while black tea leaves are richer in caffeine. It's important to pay attention to the brewing instructions for each type of tea, as over steeping or using water that is too hot can result in a bitter and unpalatable drink. Adding sweeteners such as honey, sugar or milk is a personal preference, but it's important to note that adding these can also add extra calories.

Herbal teas, on the other hand, are made from a variety of plant materials such as flowers, leaves, and roots. Unlike tea, herbal teas do not contain any caffeine and offer a variety of potential health benefits depending on the type of herb used. Chamomile, for example, is known for its calming properties, while ginger tea is often used to help with digestion. It's important to use fresh, high-quality herbs and to follow the brewing instructions carefully. Generally, herbal teas are steeped for longer than regular tea, often for up to 10 minutes, to allow the full range of flavors and health benefits to infuse into the water.

Infusions are similar to herbal teas but are typically made with more substantial ingredients such as fruits, spices, and roots. Unlike herbal tea, infusions often require a longer steeping time of up to 30 minutes to fully extract the flavor and nutrients from the ingredients. It's important to use fresh, high-quality ingredients and to experiment with different flavor combinations to find what works best for your taste buds. Popular ingredients for infusions include dried fruits like apricots and cherries, as well as spices like cinnamon and cardamom.

In summary, using the correct ingredients and brewing methods is crucial for making the perfect cup of tea, herbal tea or infusion. Take the time to experiment with different types of tea leaves, herbs, fruits, and spices to find the perfect combination of flavors and health benefits. Remember to follow brewing instructions carefully to ensure the best results.

INFUSION TIMES

Infusion time is an important factor to consider when preparing tea, herbal teas, and infusions. It can greatly affect the taste, strength, and even the health benefits of the beverage.

When it comes to tea, the recommended infusion time varies depending on the type of tea. For example, black tea should be steeped for 3-5 minutes, green tea for 1-3 minutes, and white tea for 2-3 minutes. Oolong tea typically takes 3-5 minutes, while herbal teas like chamomile or peppermint can be steeped for 5-10 minutes or even longer.

Herbal teas are made from a variety of plant materials, including leaves, flowers, roots, and berries. As such, infusion times can vary greatly depending on the specific herb being used. For instance, lavender and lemon balm should be steeped for 5-7 minutes, while ginger and echinacea require 10-15 minutes. It's important to follow instructions or recommended infusion times for each herb, as over-steeping can result in a bitter taste and potentially negate any health benefits.

Infusions, on the other hand, are made from steeping a combination of herbs, fruits, or spices in hot water. Like herbal teas, infusion times can vary greatly depending on the ingredients used. For example, an infusion of cinnamon, ginger, and lemon can be steeped for 10-15 minutes, while an infusion of rose petals and hibiscus requires only 5-7 minutes.

In general, longer infusion times result in a stronger, more flavorful beverage. However, it's important to note that over-steeping can also result in a bitter taste, and some herbs and ingredients should not be steeped for too long as it may cause a negative effect on their taste or benefits. It's best to follow the recommended infusion times for the specific type of tea, herb, or infusion you are preparing in order to get the most out of its flavor and health benefits.

THERAPEUTICAL PROPERTIES OF TEA, HERBAL TEA AND INFUSION

Tea, herbal tea, and infusion are popular beverages known for their therapeutic properties. Each of these drinks has its unique benefits, making them a popular choice for people looking to improve their overall health and wellness. In this article, we will explore the therapeutic properties of tea, herbal tea, and infusion.

Tea, which is derived from the leaves of the Camellia sinensis plant, has been consumed for centuries due to its many health benefits. Tea contains antioxidants known as catechins that have anti-inflammatory and anti-carcinogenic properties. These antioxidants help to reduce the risk of heart disease, stroke, and certain types of cancer.

Black tea, for example, is rich in theaflavins, which have been shown to reduce blood pressure and improve cholesterol levels. Green tea, on the other hand, contains a high concentration of epigallocatechin gallate (EGCG), which has been found to have cancer- fighting properties.

Herbal tea, also known as tisanes, is made from a variety of plants, including herbs, flowers, and fruits. Unlike tea, herbal tea does not come from the Camellia sinensis plant. Each herbal tea has its unique properties, and the benefits depend on the herbs used to make it.

For example, chamomile tea is known for its calming and soothing effects and is often used to help with sleep disorders and anxiety. Ginger tea is known for its anti- inflammatory properties and can help to relieve nausea and digestive issues.

Peppermint tea is known for its ability to soothe digestive issues and help with headaches.

Infusions, on the other hand, are made by steeping herbs, spices, or fruit in hot water. They are similar to herbal tea but are made by using larger quantities of the plant material and allowing it to steep for a longer time. The therapeutic properties of infusions vary depending on the ingredients used.

For example, an infusion made from lemon and ginger can help to boost the immune system and reduce inflammation. An infusion made from rose hips can help to reduce the risk of heart disease and improve the skin's appearance. An infusion made from cinnamon can help to regulate blood sugar levels and improve cognitive function.

In conclusion, tea, herbal tea, and infusion all have unique therapeutic properties that can help to improve overall health and wellness. While tea is derived from the Camellia sinensis plant, herbal tea and infusion are made from a variety of plants and herbs.

Understanding the therapeutic properties of these beverages can help you choose the right one to suit your needs.

Chapter 2

33 HOME RECIPES

1. Red Apple Tea

Ingredients:

- 2 red apples

- 4 cups of water

- 2 cinnamon sticks

- 1 tablespoon honey

Instructions:

- Wash the apples thoroughly and cut them into thin slices.

- In a pot, bring 4 cups of water to a boil.

- Add the sliced apples and cinnamon sticks to the pot and reduce heat to a simmer.

- Allow the mixture to simmer for 20-25 minutes or until the apples are soft and the water turns slightly red.

- Remove from heat and strain the mixture into a pitcher or teapot.

- Add honey to taste.

- Serve hot and enjoy!

Note: Alternatively, you can use store-bought apple tea bags and simply add a few slices of fresh red apple and cinnamon to enhance the flavor. Simply steep the apple tea bags in boiling water, add the apple slices and cinnamon, and allow to steep for 5-10 minutes before removing the tea bags and serving hot.

2. Coconut and Pineapple Tea

Ingredients:

- 4 cups water

- 4 tea bags

- 1 cup unsweetened pineapple juice

- 1/2 cup coconut milk

- 2 tbsp honey

Instructions:

- In a medium saucepan, bring water to a boil.

- Remove from heat and add tea bags. Steep for 3-5 minutes.

- Remove tea bags and stir in pineapple juice, coconut milk, and honey.

- Return the pan to the stove and heat on medium-low for a few minutes until heated through.

- Serve hot and enjoy!

3. Strawberry and Cardamom Tea

Ingredients:

- 1 cup sliced fresh strawberries

- 1/2 tsp ground cardamom

- 2 black tea bags

- 4 cups water

- Honey or sugar (optional)

Instructions:

- In a medium saucepan, combine the sliced strawberries, ground cardamom, and water.

- Bring the mixture to a boil over medium heat, then reduce the heat to low and simmer for 5-10 minutes.

- Add the black tea bags and steep for 3-5 minutes, depending on how strong you like your tea.

- Remove the tea bags and strain the tea through a fine-mesh strainer or cheesecloth to remove any solids.

- Serve hot, sweetened with honey or sugar if desired.

- If you prefer iced tea, let the mixture cool and serve over ice.

- Enjoy your refreshing and flavorful Strawberry and Cardamom Tea!

4. Red Fruit and Cinnamon Tea

Ingredients:

- 1/2 cup mixed red berries (such as raspberries, strawberries, and cranberries)

- 1 cinnamon stick

- 2 black tea bags

- 4 cups water

- Honey or sugar (optional)

Instructions:

- In a medium saucepan, combine the mixed red berries, cinnamon stick, and water.

- Bring the mixture to a boil over medium heat, then reduce the heat to low and simmer for 5-10 minutes.

- Add the black tea bags and steep for 3-5 minutes, depending on how strong you like your tea.

- Remove the tea bags and cinnamon stick and strain the tea through a fine-mesh strainer or cheesecloth to remove any solids.

- Serve hot, sweetened with honey or sugar if desired.

- If you prefer iced tea, let the mixture cool and serve over ice.

- Enjoy your delicious and fruity Red Fruit and Cinnamon Tea!

5. Black Pepper Tea

Ingredients:

- 2 cups of water

- 1 tsp black tea leaves

- 1 tsp honey

- 1/4 tsp black pepper

- 1/4 tsp grated ginger

- 1/4 tsp cinnamon powder

- 1/4 tsp cardamom powder

- 1/4 tsp clove powder

- 1/4 tsp fennel seeds

- 1/4 tsp cumin seeds

- 1/4 tsp coriander seeds

Instructions:

- In a saucepan, bring 2 cups of water to a boil.

- Add the black tea leaves to the boiling water and let it steep for 2-3 minutes.

- Meanwhile, grind the black pepper, ginger, cinnamon powder, cardamom powder, clove powder, fennel seeds, cumin seeds, and coriander seeds together in a mortar and pestle.

- Add the spice mixture to the tea and stir well.

- Let the tea simmer for 2-3 minutes on low heat.

- Strain the tea and add honey to taste.

- Serve hot and enjoy the warm, spicy flavors of black pepper tea.

Note: You can adjust the quantity of black pepper according to your taste preferences. If you prefer a milder flavor, use less black pepper. You can also add milk or cream to make the tea creamier and more indulgent. This tea can help soothe a sore throat, ease congestion, and aid digestion. It's best to consume this tea in moderation and consult a healthcare professional before adding it to your diet if you have any medical conditions or allergies.

6. Chocolate Banana Tea

Ingredients:

- 2 cups water

- 1 banana, mashed

- 1 tablespoon unsweetened cocoa powder

- 1 tablespoon honey

- 1 cinnamon stick

- 1 tea bag (black tea or chai tea)

Instructions:

- In a small saucepan, bring 2 cups of water to a boil.

- Add the mashed banana, unsweetened cocoa powder, honey, and cinnamon stick to the boiling water. Stir well and reduce heat to medium.

- Let the mixture simmer for 5-7 minutes, stirring occasionally, until the banana is fully cooked and the mixture thickens slightly.

- Remove the cinnamon stick and add a tea bag to the mixture. Let it steep for 2-3 minutes.

- Remove the tea bag and strain the mixture through a fine-mesh sieve to remove any banana solids.

- Serve hot and enjoy the delicious combination of chocolate and banana in your tea.

Note: You can use black tea or chai tea for this recipe, depending on your preference. If you want a smoother texture, you can blend the mixture in a blender or use an immersion blender. You can adjust the sweetness level by adding more or less honey. This tea is a great way to indulge your sweet tooth while still enjoying the benefits of tea. It's best to consume this tea in moderation and consult a healthcare professional before adding it to your diet if you have any medical conditions or allergies.

7. Milk Tea with Saffron and Honey

Ingredients:

- 2 cups water

- 1 black tea bag (or 2 tsps loose black tea leaves)

- 1/4 tsp saffron threads

- 2 tablespoons honey (adjust to taste)

- 1 cup milk (any type of milk, such as whole milk, almond milk, or coconut milk)

- 1 cinnamon stick (optional)

Instructions:

- In a small saucepan, bring 2 cups of water to a boil.

- Add the black tea bag (or loose tea leaves) to the boiling water and let it steep for 3-5 minutes.

- Meanwhile, crush the saffron threads using a mortar and pestle.

- Add the crushed saffron threads to the tea and stir well.

- Add honey to the tea and stir until fully dissolved.

- Add milk to the tea and let it simmer on low heat for 5-7 minutes, stirring occasionally.

- If using, add a cinnamon stick to the tea and let it simmer for an additional minute.

- Strain the tea through a fine-mesh sieve to remove any tea leaves, saffron threads, or cinnamon stick.

- Serve hot and enjoy the creamy, fragrant, and slightly sweet flavors of saffron and honey milk tea.

Note: Saffron can be expensive, but a little goes a long way in this recipe. You can also substitute saffron with turmeric for a more affordable option. You can adjust the sweetness level by adding more or less honey. This tea is a great way to add a unique and exotic twist to your regular milk tea. It's best to consume this tea in moderation and consult a healthcare professional before adding it to your diet if you have any medical conditions or allergies.

8. Lemon and Bergamot Tea

Ingredients:

- 2 cups water

- 1 black tea bag (or 2 tsps loose black tea leaves)

- 1/4 tsp dried bergamot leaves (or 1-2 drops of bergamot essential oil)

- 1 lemon, thinly sliced

- 2 tablespoons honey (adjust to taste)

Instructions:

- In a small saucepan, bring 2 cups of water to a boil.

- Add the black tea bag (or loose tea leaves) to the boiling water and let it steep for 3-5 minutes.

- Meanwhile, crush the dried bergamot leaves using a mortar and pestle.

- Add the crushed bergamot leaves to the tea and stir well.

- Add thinly sliced lemon to the tea and stir

- Add honey to the tea and stir until fully dissolved.

- Let the tea simmer on low heat for 5-7 minutes, stirring occasionally.

- Strain the tea through a fine-mesh sieve to remove any tea leaves or bergamot leaves.

- Serve hot and enjoy the refreshing, citrusy, and floral flavors of lemon and bergamot tea.

Note: Bergamot leaves can be difficult to find, but you can substitute them with bergamot essential oil. Use 1-2 drops of bergamot essential oil in the tea, depending on your preference. You can adjust the sweetness level by adding more or less honey. This tea is a great way to enjoy the combined flavors of lemon and bergamot, which complement each other perfectly. It's best to consume this tea in moderation and consult a healthcare professional before adding it to your diet if you have any medical conditions or allergies.

9. Grapefruit and Pomegranate Tea

Ingredients:

- 2 cups water

- 1 grapefruit, cut into wedges

- 1/2 cup pomegranate arils

- 1 tablespoon honey (adjust to taste)

- 2 black tea bags (or 4 tsps loose black tea leaves

Instructions:

- In a small saucepan, bring 2 cups of water to a boil.

- Add the grapefruit wedges to the boiling water and let them steep for 3-5 minutes.

- Meanwhile, add the pomegranate arils to a blender and blend until they are roughly chopped.

- Remove the grapefruit wedges from the water and add the black tea bags (or loose tea leaves) to the water.

- Let the tea steep for 3-5 minutes

- Remove the tea bags (or strain the loose tea leaves).

- Add the chopped pomegranate arils to the tea and stir well.

- Add honey to the tea and stir until fully dissolved.

- Serve hot or chilled, and enjoy the tangy, fruity, and slightly sweet flavors of grapefruit and pomegranate tea.

Note: This tea is a great way to enjoy the health benefits of both grapefruit and pomegranate, which are rich in antioxidants and vitamins. You can also garnish the tea with additional pomegranate arils or grapefruit wedges for a more visually appealing presentation.

10. Star Anise Tea with Milk and Vanilla

Ingredients:

- 4 cups water

- 4 whole star anise pods

- 2 cinnamon sticks

- 1 vanilla bean, split lengthwise

- 2 cups milk (or dairy-free milk substitute)

- 2 tablespoons honey (adjust to taste)

Instructions:

- In a large saucepan, bring 4 cups of water to a boil.

- Add the star anise pods and cinnamon sticks to the boiling water and let them steep for 5-7 minutes.

- Scrape the seeds out of the vanilla bean using a knife and add them to the tea. Then, add the split vanilla bean to the tea as well.

- Let the tea simmer on low heat for 10-15 minutes, stirring occasionally.

- Add milk to the tea and stir well.

- Add honey to the tea and stir until fully dissolved.

- Let the tea simmer for an additional 5-7 minutes, stirring occasionally.

- Remove the vanilla bean, star anise pods, and cinnamon sticks from the tea using a slotted spoon.

- Serve hot and enjoy the rich, creamy, and slightly sweet flavors of star anise tea with milk and vanilla.

Note: You can adjust the sweetness level by adding more or less honey. This tea is a great way to enjoy the unique flavor of star anise, which has a licorice-like taste and is commonly used in Asian cuisine. If you don't have a vanilla bean, you can substitute it with 1 tsp of vanilla extract. You can use any type of milk or dairy-free milk substitute that you prefer, such as almond milk, coconut milk, or soy milk. This tea can be served as a dessert drink or a warming treat on a chilly day.

11. Milk Tea with Vanilla and Banana

Ingredients:

- 4 cups water

- 4 black tea bags (or 4 tsps loose black tea leaves)

- 2 ripe bananas, mashed

- 1 vanilla bean, split lengthwise

- 2 cups milk (or dairy-free milk substitute)

- 2 tablespoons honey (adjust to taste)

Instructions:

- In a large saucepan, bring 4 cups of water to a boil.

- Add the black tea bags (or loose tea leaves) to the boiling water and let them steep for 3-5 minutes.

- Meanwhile, in a separate bowl, mash the bananas until they are smooth and free of lumps.

- Scrape the seeds out of the vanilla bean using a knife and add them to the tea. Then, add the split vanilla bean to the tea as well.

- Add the mashed bananas to the tea and stir well.

- Let the tea simmer on low heat for 10-15 minutes, stirring occasionally.

- Add milk to the tea and stir well.

- Add honey to the tea and stir until fully dissolved.

- Let the tea simmer for an additional 5-7 minutes, stirring occasionally.

- Remove the vanilla bean from the tea using a slotted spoon.

- Serve hot and enjoy the creamy, fruity, and slightly sweet flavors of milk tea with vanilla and banana.

Note: You can adjust the sweetness level by adding more or less honey. This tea is a great way to enjoy the natural sweetness of bananas, which are a good source of vitamins and fiber. If you don't have a vanilla bean, you can substitute it with 1 tsp of vanilla extract. You can use any type of milk or dairy-free milk substitute that you prefer, such as almond milk, coconut milk, or soy milk. This tea can be served as a dessert drink or a comforting treat on a lazy afternoon.

12. Dandelion Herbal Tea

Ingredients:

- 4 cups water

- 2 tablespoons dried dandelion root

- 2 tablespoons dried dandelion leaves

- 1 cinnamon stick

- 1 tsp honey (adjust to taste)

- Juice of half a lemon (optional)

Instructions:

- In a large saucepan, bring 4 cups of water to a boil.

- Add the dried dandelion root and leaves to the boiling water and let them steep for 5-7 minutes.

- Add the cinnamon stick to the tea and let it steep for an additional 2-3 minutes.

- Remove the tea from the heat and let it cool for a few minutes.

- Add honey to the tea and stir until fully dissolved.

- If desired, add the juice of half a lemon to the tea and stir well.

- Strain the tea through a fine mesh strainer into a teapot or individual cups.

- Serve hot and enjoy the earthy, slightly bitter, and warming flavors of dandelion herbal tea.

Note: Dandelion root and leaves are commonly used in herbal medicine and are believed to have a number of health benefits, such as improving digestion and liver function. If you don't have dried dandelion root and leaves, you can use fresh ones. Simply wash them well and chop them into small pieces before adding them to the tea. You can adjust the sweetness level by adding more or less honey. You can also add other herbs or spices to the tea, such as ginger, cardamom, or clove, to enhance the flavor and aroma. Dandelion herbal tea can be enjoyed any time of the day, but it is especially nice to sip in the evening or before bed as it can help to promote relaxation and sleep.

13. Birch Herbal Tea

Ingredients:

- 4 cups water

- 2 tablespoons dried birch leaves

- 1 tablespoon dried chamomile flowers

- 1 tablespoon honey (adjust to taste)

- Juice of half a lemon (optional)

Instructions:

- In a large saucepan, bring 4 cups of water to a boil.

- Add the dried birch leaves to the boiling water and let them steep for 5-7 minutes.

- Add the dried chamomile flowers to the tea and let them steep for an additional 2- 3 minutes.

- Remove the tea from the heat and let it cool for a few minutes.

- Add honey to the tea and stir until fully dissolved.

- If desired, add the juice of half a lemon to the tea and stir well.

- Strain the tea through a fine mesh strainer into a teapot or individual cups.

- Serve hot and enjoy the refreshing, floral, and slightly sweet flavors of birch herbal tea.

Note: Birch leaves are commonly used in traditional medicine and are believed to have anti-inflammatory and diuretic properties. Chamomile flowers are also known for their calming and soothing effects, making this tea a great choice for relaxation and stress relief. If you don't have dried birch leaves, you can use fresh ones. Simply wash them well and chop them into small pieces before adding them to the tea. You can adjust the sweetness level by adding more or less honey. Birch herbal tea can be enjoyed any time of the day, but it is especially nice to sip in the afternoon or evening as it can help to promote relaxation and calmness.

14. Parsley and Lime Herbal Tea

Ingredients:

- 4 cups water

- 1 cup fresh parsley leaves

- 1 lime, sliced

- 1 tablespoon honey (adjust to taste)

Instructions:

- In a large saucepan, bring 4 cups of water to a boil.

- Add the fresh parsley leaves to the boiling water and let them steep for 5-7 minutes.

- Remove the parsley leaves from the tea and discard.

- Add the sliced lime to the tea and let it steep for an additional 2-3 minutes.

- Remove the tea from the heat and let it cool for a few minutes.

- Add honey to the tea and stir until fully dissolved.

- Strain the tea through a fine mesh strainer into a teapot or individual cups.

- Serve hot or iced and enjoy the refreshing and tangy flavors of parsley and lime herbal tea.

Note: Parsley is a rich source of antioxidants, vitamins, and minerals and is believed to have a number of health benefits, such as improving digestion and boosting the immune system. Lime is also rich in vitamin C and has a refreshing and tangy flavor that pairs well with parsley. Parsley and lime herbal tea can be enjoyed any time of the day, but it is especially nice to sip in the morning as it can help to promote detoxification and boost energy levels. You can also add other herbs or spices to the tea, such as ginger or mint, to enhance the flavor and aroma.

15. Yerba Mate herbal mate

Ingredients:

- 1/4 cup of Yerba Mate leaves

- 2 cups of hot water

- Optional: honey, lemon, or mint

Instructions:

- Heat the water to just before boiling.

- Place the Yerba Mate leaves in a tea strainer or tea bag.

- Pour the hot water over the Yerba Mate leaves and let it steep for 3-5 minutes.

- Remove the tea strainer or tea bag and discard the leaves.

- If desired, add honey, lemon, or mint for flavor.

- Serve hot and enjoy!

Note: Yerba Mate is a traditional South American beverage that's said to have numerous health benefits, including boosting energy, improving mental clarity, and aiding digestion. This herbal mate is a great way to enjoy those benefits in a tasty and easy-to-make drink. Enjoy it as a morning pick-me-up or an afternoon refreshment.

16. Turmeric and Cumin Herbal Tea

Ingredients:

- 4 cups water

- 1 tablespoon ground turmeric

- 1 tsp ground cumin

- 1 cinnamon stick

- 1 tablespoon honey (adjust to taste)

- Juice of half a lemon (optional)

Instructions:

- In a large saucepan, bring 4 cups of water to a boil.

- Add the ground turmeric, ground cumin, and cinnamon stick to the boiling water and let them steep for 5-7 minutes.

- Remove the tea from the heat and let it cool for a few minutes.

- Add honey to the tea and stir until fully dissolved.

- If desired, add the juice of half a lemon to the tea and stir well.

- Strain the tea through a fine mesh strainer into a teapot or individual cups.

- Serve hot and enjoy the warm and earthy flavors of turmeric and cumin herbal tea.

Note: Turmeric and cumin are both known for their anti-inflammatory and antioxidant properties, making this tea a great choice for promoting overall health and wellness. Cinnamon adds a subtle sweetness and warmth to the tea, while honey provides a natural sweetener. If you prefer a stronger tea, you can increase the amount of turmeric and cumin used. Turmeric and cumin herbal tea can be enjoyed any time of the day, but it is especially nice to sip in the evening as it can help to promote relaxation and reduce stress levels. You can also add other spices to the tea, such as ginger or black pepper, to enhance the flavor and aroma.

17. Tisana al cardo Mariano e cumino

Ingredients:

- 4 cups of water

- 1 tablespoon of milk thistle seeds

- 1 tsp of cumin seeds

- 1 cinnamon stick

- 1 tablespoon honey (adjust to taste)

Instructions:

- In a large pot, bring 4 cups of water to a boil.

- Add the milk thistle seeds, cumin seeds and cinnamon stick to the boiling water and let them steep for 5-7 minutes.

- Remove the herbal tea from the heat and let it cool for a few minutes.

- Add the honey to the herbal tea and stir until completely dissolved.

- Strain the herbal tea through a fine mesh strainer into individual teapots or cups.

- Serve hot and enjoy the rich, earthy flavors of Milk Thistle Cumin Tea.

Note: Milk thistle and cumin are known for their digestive and antioxidant properties, making this herbal tea a great choice for supporting the health of the gastrointestinal tract. The cinnamon adds a subtle sweetness and warmth to the herbal tea, while the honey provides a natural sweetener. If you prefer a stronger herbal tea, you can increase the amount of milk thistle and cumin seeds you use. Milk thistle and cumin herbal tea can be enjoyed at any time of the day, but it is particularly pleasant to sip after meals to aid digestion. You can also add other spices to the herbal tea, such as ginger or black pepper, to enrich the flavor and aroma.

18. Dandelion, Mint, and Turmeric Herbal Tea

Ingredients:

- 4 cups water

- 1 tablespoon dried dandelion root

- 1 tsp dried turmeric root or powder

- 1/4 cup fresh mint leaves, roughly chopped

- 1 tablespoon honey (optional)

Instructions:

- In a large pot, bring 4 cups of water to a boil.

- Add the dried dandelion root and turmeric to the boiling water and let it simmer for about 5 minutes.

- Turn off the heat and add the fresh mint leaves to the pot. Let it steep for an additional 5 minutes.

- Strain the tea through a fine-mesh sieve into a teapot or individual cups.

- Add honey, if desired, to sweeten the tea to your liking.

- Serve the tea hot and enjoy the refreshing taste and health benefits of dandelion, mint, and turmeric.

Note: Dandelion root is known for its detoxifying properties, while turmeric is known for its anti-inflammatory properties. Together, they make a powerful herbal tea that promotes overall health and wellness. Mint adds a refreshing flavor and aroma to the tea and also aids in digestion. This tea can be enjoyed any time of day, but is especially nice to drink in the morning or after a meal. To enhance the flavor and health benefits, you can add a slice of fresh ginger or a pinch of black pepper to the tea. If you don't have access to fresh mint leaves, you can use 1 tablespoon of dried mint instead.

19. Herbal Tea with Cloves and Dried Figs

Ingredients:

- 4 cups water

- 4 dried figs

- 1 cinnamon stick

- 2 whole cloves

- 2 tea bags of your choice (black tea or herbal tea)

- Honey or sugar (optional)

Instructions:

- In a medium-sized pot, bring 4 cups of water to a boil.

- Add the dried figs, cinnamon stick, and cloves to the pot.

- Let the mixture simmer for 10-15 minutes, until the water has turned a rich, dark color.

- Remove the pot from heat and add the tea bags of your choice.

- Let the tea bags steep for 3-5 minutes, depending on your desired strength.

- Remove the tea bags and strain the tea through a fine-mesh sieve to remove the dried figs and spices.

- Serve hot, optionally sweetened with honey or sugar to taste.

Note: This tea is perfect for colder months or as a soothing drink before bedtime. Dried figs add natural sweetness to the tea, while cloves and cinnamon give it a warm and spicy flavor. You can also add other spices like cardamom or nutmeg for more depth of flavor. You can use either black tea or herbal tea for this recipe, depending on your preference. The tea can be stored in the fridge for up to 3 days and reheated as needed.

20. Wild Fennel Herbal Tea

Ingredients:

- 4 cups water

- 1/2 cup wild fennel fronds, chopped

- 1 lemon, sliced

- Honey or sugar (optional)

Instructions:

- In a medium-sized pot, bring 4 cups of water to a boil.

- Add the chopped wild fennel fronds to the pot and let it simmer for 5-7 minutes.

- Turn off the heat and add the lemon slices to the pot.

- Let the tea steep for an additional 5-10 minutes.

- Strain the tea through a fine-mesh sieve into a teapot or individual cups.

- Add honey or sugar, if desired, to sweeten the tea to your liking.

- Serve the tea hot and enjoy the refreshing taste and health benefits of wild fennel.

Note: Wild fennel is known for its many health benefits, including improved digestion and respiratory health. The lemon slices add a bright and tangy flavor to the tea and also provide additional health benefits. This tea is caffeine-free and can be enjoyed at any time of the day. You can also add other herbs like mint or chamomile to the tea for added flavor and benefits. Wild fennel can be found in many areas throughout the world, but if you cannot find it, you can use regular fennel fronds instead.

21. Mint and Mallow Herbal Tea

Ingredients:

- 4 cups water

- 1/2 cup fresh mint leaves, chopped

- 1/4 cup dried mallow flowers

- Honey or sugar (optional)

Instructions:

- In a medium-sized pot, bring 4 cups of water to a boil.

- Add the chopped fresh mint leaves and dried mallow flowers to the pot.

- Let the mixture simmer for 5-7 minutes, until the water has turned a light green color.

- Turn off the heat and let the tea steep for an additional 5-10 minutes.

- Strain the tea through a fine-mesh sieve into a teapot or individual cups.

- Add honey or sugar, if desired, to sweeten the tea to your liking.

- Serve the tea hot and enjoy the refreshing taste and health benefits of mint and mallow.

Note: Mint and mallow are both known for their many health benefits, including improved digestion and respiratory health. Mallow flowers add a sweet and floral flavor to the tea, while mint leaves provide a refreshing and cooling effect. This tea is caffeine- free and can be enjoyed at any time of the day. You can also add other herbs like lemon balm or chamomile to the tea for added flavor and benefits. If you cannot find fresh mint leaves, you can use dried mint leaves instead.

22. Lemongrass Herbal Tea

Ingredients:

- 4 cups water

- 1 stalk of lemongrass, chopped

- 1 tsp honey (optional)

- 1 lemon slice (optional)

Instructions:

- In a medium-sized pot, bring 4 cups of water to a boil.

- Add the chopped lemongrass to the pot and let it simmer for 5-7 minutes.

- Turn off the heat and let the tea steep for an additional 5-10 minutes.

- Strain the tea through a fine-mesh sieve into a teapot or individual cups.

- Add honey, if desired, to sweeten the tea to your liking.

- For an extra zesty flavor, add a lemon slice to the tea.

- Serve the tea hot and enjoy the refreshing taste and health benefits of lemongrass.

Note: Lemongrass is known for its many health benefits, including improved digestion and immune system function. This tea is caffeine-free and can be enjoyed at any time of the day. You can also add other herbs like ginger or mint to the tea for added flavor and benefits. If you can't find fresh lemongrass, you can use dried lemongrass instead, but use only half the amount. Make sure to wash the lemongrass thoroughly before using it in the tea.

23. Cardamom and Dried Figs Infusion

Ingredients:

- 4 cups water

- 8 green cardamom pods, crushed

- 4 dried figs, sliced

- 1 tsp honey (optional)

Instructions:

- In a medium-sized pot, bring 4 cups of water to a boil.

- Add the crushed cardamom pods to the pot and let them simmer for 5-7 minutes.

- Add the dried figs to the pot and let them simmer for an additional 5-7 minutes.

- Turn off the heat and let the infusion steep for an additional 5-10 minutes.

- Strain the infusion through a fine-mesh sieve into a teapot or individual cups.

- Add honey, if desired, to sweeten the infusion to your liking.

- Serve the infusion hot and enjoy the warm and comforting flavors of cardamom and dried figs.

Note: Cardamom is known for its many health benefits, including improved digestion and detoxification. Dried figs are a good source of fiber, antioxidants, and other important nutrients. This infusion is caffeine-free and can be enjoyed at any time of the day. You can also add other spices like cinnamon or ginger to the infusion for added flavor and benefits. Make sure to crush the cardamom pods to release their flavorful oils before adding them to the pot. Use only dried figs for this recipe, as fresh figs will not hold up well in the infusion.

24. Ginger Infusion

Ingredients:

- 4 cups water

- 2-3 inches fresh ginger root, peeled and sliced

- 1 tablespoon honey (optional)

- Juice of 1/2 lemon (optional)

Instructions:

- In a medium-sized pot, bring 4 cups of water to a boil.

- Add the sliced ginger to the pot and let it simmer for 10-15 minutes.

- Turn off the heat and let the infusion steep for an additional 5-10 minutes.

- Strain the infusion through a fine-mesh sieve into a teapot or individual cups.

- Add honey and/or lemon juice, if desired, to sweeten and enhance the flavor of the infusion.

- Serve the infusion hot and enjoy the warming and invigorating flavors of fresh ginger.

Note: Ginger is known for its many health benefits, including reducing inflammation, improving digestion, and boosting the immune system. This infusion is caffeine-free and can be enjoyed at any time of the day. You can adjust the amount of ginger used in the recipe depending on your personal preference for spiciness. To store any leftover ginger infusion, let it cool to room temperature before transferring it to an airtight container and refrigerating it for up to 3 days. This infusion can also be enjoyed cold by letting it cool to room temperature before transferring it to a pitcher and refrigerating it for a few hours or overnight. Serve over ice and enjoy the refreshing and zesty flavors of ginger.

25. Watermelon and Basil Infusion

Ingredients:

- 4 cups of water

- 4 cups of watermelon chunks

- 4-6 fresh basil leaves

- 1 tablespoon honey (optional)

- Juice of 1/2 lime (optional)

Instructions:

- In a blender, puree the watermelon chunks until they become a smooth liquid.

- In a medium-sized pot, bring 4 cups of water to a boil.

- Add the basil leaves to the pot and let it simmer for 5-10 minutes.

- Turn off the heat and let the basil infusion steep for an additional 5-10 minutes.

- Strain the basil infusion through a fine-mesh sieve into a pitcher.

- Add the watermelon puree to the pitcher and stir well.

- Add honey and/or lime juice, if desired, to sweeten and enhance the flavor of the infusion.

- Let the infusion cool to room temperature, then refrigerate for at least 1 hour or until chilled.

- Serve the infusion over ice and garnish with additional basil leaves and watermelon chunks, if desired.

Note: Watermelon is a great source of hydration and is rich in vitamins A and C, while basil adds a refreshing and aromatic flavor to the infusion. This infusion is caffeine-free and can be enjoyed at any time of the day. You can adjust the amount of honey and lime juice used in the recipe depending on your personal preference for sweetness and acidity. To store any leftover watermelon and basil infusion, let it cool to room temperature before transferring it to an airtight container and refrigerating it for up to 3 days. This infusion can also be enjoyed as a cocktail by adding a splash of your favorite liquor, such as vodka or gin, for a refreshing summer drink.

26. Cucumber and Mint Infusion

Ingredients:

- 1 large cucumber, peeled and sliced

- 6-8 fresh mint leaves

- 4 cups of water

- 1 tablespoon honey (optional)

- Juice of 1/2 lime (optional)

- Ice cubes, for serving

Instructions:

- In a large pitcher, add the sliced cucumber and fresh mint leaves.

- Using a muddler or wooden spoon, muddle the cucumber and mint together until the cucumber is slightly broken down and the mint leaves are fragrant.

- Pour 4 cups of water into the pitcher and stir well.

- Cover the pitcher and let it sit in the refrigerator for at least 2 hours or overnight to infuse.

- Before serving, stir the infusion well and taste. If desired, add honey and/or lime juice to sweeten and enhance the flavor.

- Serve the infusion over ice cubes and garnish with additional cucumber slices and mint leaves, if desired.

Note: Cucumber is a refreshing and hydrating fruit that is low in calories and high in vitamins and minerals, while mint adds a refreshing and aromatic flavor to the infusion. This infusion is caffeine-free and can be enjoyed at any time of the day. You can adjust the amount of honey and lime juice used in the recipe depending on your personal preference for sweetness and acidity. To store any leftover cucumber and mint infusion, let it cool to room temperature before transferring it to an airtight container and refrigerating it for up to 3 days. This infusion can also be used as a base for cocktails by adding a splash of your favorite liquor, such as gin or vodka, for a refreshing summer drink

27. Lemon and Pink Pepper Infusion

Ingredients:

- 4 cups water

- 1 lemon, sliced

- 1 tablespoon pink peppercorns

- 2 tablespoons honey (optional)

Instructions:

- In a medium-sized saucepan, bring 4 cups of water to a boil.

- Once the water has come to a boil, remove it from heat and add the sliced lemon and pink peppercorns.

- Let the mixture steep for 10-15 minutes, or until the flavors have fully infused.

- Strain the liquid into a pitcher, using a fine mesh strainer to remove the lemon slices and peppercorns.

- If desired, stir in honey until it dissolves and adjust the sweetness to your liking.

- Serve the infusion warm or chill in the refrigerator for 1-2 hours before serving over ice.

Note: The combination of lemon and pink pepper creates a unique and refreshing flavor that is both tangy and slightly spicy. Pink peppercorns are not actually related to black pepper and have a more subtle flavor with a slight sweetness. This infusion is a great alternative to caffeinated beverages like coffee or tea and can be enjoyed at any time of the day. The addition of honey is optional and can be adjusted according to your taste preference. This infusion can also be used as a base for cocktails by adding a splash of your favorite liquor, such as gin or vodka, for a delicious and refreshing drink. Leftover infusion can be stored in the refrigerator for up to 3 days in an airtight container.

28. Infusion of Cinnamon and Cloves

Ingredients:

- 2 cinnamon sticks

- 1 tablespoon of whole cloves

- 4 cups of water

- Honey or sweetener (optional)

Instructions:

- In a small saucepan, bring the water to a boil.

- Add the cinnamon sticks and cloves to the boiling water.

- Reduce the heat to low and let the mixture simmer for about 15-20 minutes. This will allow the flavors of cinnamon and cloves to infuse into the water.

- After simmering, remove the saucepan from heat and let it cool slightly.

- Strain the infusion using a fine-mesh sieve or a tea strainer to remove the cinnamon sticks and cloves.

- If desired, add honey or sweetener to taste, stirring until it dissolves completely.

- Pour the infused cinnamon and cloves into cups or mugs.

- Serve the infusion hot and enjoy its comforting flavors.

Note: You can adjust the quantity of cinnamon sticks and cloves based on your preference for a stronger or milder flavor. Additionally, feel free to experiment with other spices or add citrus peels for variations in taste.

29. Orange and Lime Infusion

Ingredients:

- 4 cups of water

- 1 orange, sliced

- 1 lime, sliced

- 1 tablespoon of honey (optional)

- Fresh mint leaves (optional)

Instructions:

- In a large pot, bring 4 cups of water to a boil.

- Add the sliced orange and lime to the pot and stir.

- Reduce the heat to low and let the mixture simmer for 10-15 minutes.

- Remove the pot from the heat and let it cool for a few minutes.

- Strain the liquid into a pitcher, removing the fruit slices and any seeds or pulp.

- If desired, stir in honey until it dissolves and adjust the sweetness to your liking.

- Add fresh mint leaves for an extra burst of flavor.

- Chill the infusion in the refrigerator for at least 1 hour before serving over ice.

Note: This infusion is a great way to hydrate and refresh yourself during hot summer days. The combination of orange and lime provides a tangy, citrusy flavor that is perfectly balanced. The addition of honey is optional and can be adjusted according to your taste preference. Mint leaves add a refreshing twist to the infusion and can be used as a garnish as well. Leftover infusion can be stored in the refrigerator for up to 3 days in an airtight container. This infusion can also be used as a base for cocktails. Simply add a splash of your favorite liquor, such as rum or vodka, for an adult version of the drink.

30. Blueberry and Pineapple Infusion

Ingredients:

- 4 cups of water

- 1 cup of blueberries

- 1 cup of pineapple chunks

- 1 tablespoon of honey (optional)

- Fresh mint leaves (optional)

Instructions:

- In a large pot, bring 4 cups of water to a boil.

- Add the blueberries and pineapple chunks to the pot and stir.

- Reduce the heat to low and let the mixture simmer for 10-15 minutes.

- Remove the pot from the heat and let it cool for a few minutes.

- Strain the liquid into a pitcher, removing the fruit pieces and any seeds or pulp.

- If desired, stir in honey until it dissolves and adjust the sweetness to your liking.

- Add fresh mint leaves for an extra burst of flavor.

- Chill the infusion in the refrigerator for at least 1 hour before serving over ice.

Note: This infusion is a great way to enjoy the sweetness of blueberries and pineapples in a refreshing drink. The combination of blueberries and pineapples provides a balance of sweet and tart flavors. The addition of honey is optional and can be adjusted according to your taste preference. Mint leaves add a refreshing twist to the infusion and can be used as a garnish as well. Leftover infusion can be stored in the refrigerator for up to 3 days in an airtight container. This infusion can also be used as a base for cocktails. Simply add a splash of your favorite liquor, such as rum or vodka, for an adult version of the drink.

31. Strawberry and Bergamot Infusion

Ingredients:

- 1 cup sliced strawberries

- 1 bergamot orange, sliced

- 4 cups water

- Honey, to taste

Instructions:

- In a saucepan, bring water to a boil.

- Add the sliced strawberries and bergamot orange to the boiling water.

- Let it simmer for 10-15 minutes, stirring occasionally.

- Remove from heat and let the mixture cool for a few minutes.

- Strain the mixture and pour the infused water into a pitcher.

- Add honey to taste and stir well.

- Chill in the refrigerator for at least an hour.

- Serve over ice and enjoy your refreshing strawberry and bergamot infusion.

Note: You can also add some fresh mint leaves or a squeeze of lime to add an extra kick to this infusion.

32. Pear and Vanilla Infusion

Ingredients:

- 2 ripe pears, sliced

- 4 cups of water

- 1 vanilla bean, split lengthwise

- Honey (optional)

Instructions:

- In a pot, add the sliced pears and water. Bring it to a boil over medium-high heat.

- Reduce the heat to low and let it simmer for about 20 minutes, until the pears become soft.

- Turn off the heat and add the vanilla bean to the pot. Let it steep for 10 minutes.

- Remove the vanilla bean and discard it. Using a strainer, strain the pear and vanilla mixture into a pitcher or teapot.

- If you prefer a sweeter taste, you can add honey to the infusion.

- Serve the pear and vanilla infusion hot or let it cool in the refrigerator for a refreshing iced tea.

- Enjoy the delicate sweetness of pears and the warm aroma of vanilla in this comforting and soothing infusion.

33. Infusion of Wild Berries and Cherries

Ingredients:

- 1 cup mixed wild berries (such as blackberries, raspberries, and blueberries)

- 1 cup cherries, pitted and halved

- 4 cups water

- 2 cinnamon sticks

- 1 tsp vanilla extract

- 1 tbsp honey (optional)

Instructions:

- In a large saucepan, bring the water to a boil.

- Add the mixed wild berries, cherries, and cinnamon sticks to the saucepan.

- Reduce heat and let the mixture simmer for 10-15 minutes.

- Remove from heat and strain the mixture through a fine mesh strainer or cheesecloth into a teapot.

Stir in the vanilla extract and honey (if using) until well combined.

Serve hot or chilled.

Enjoy the delicious infusion of wild berries and cherries as a refreshing and healthy drink any time of the day!

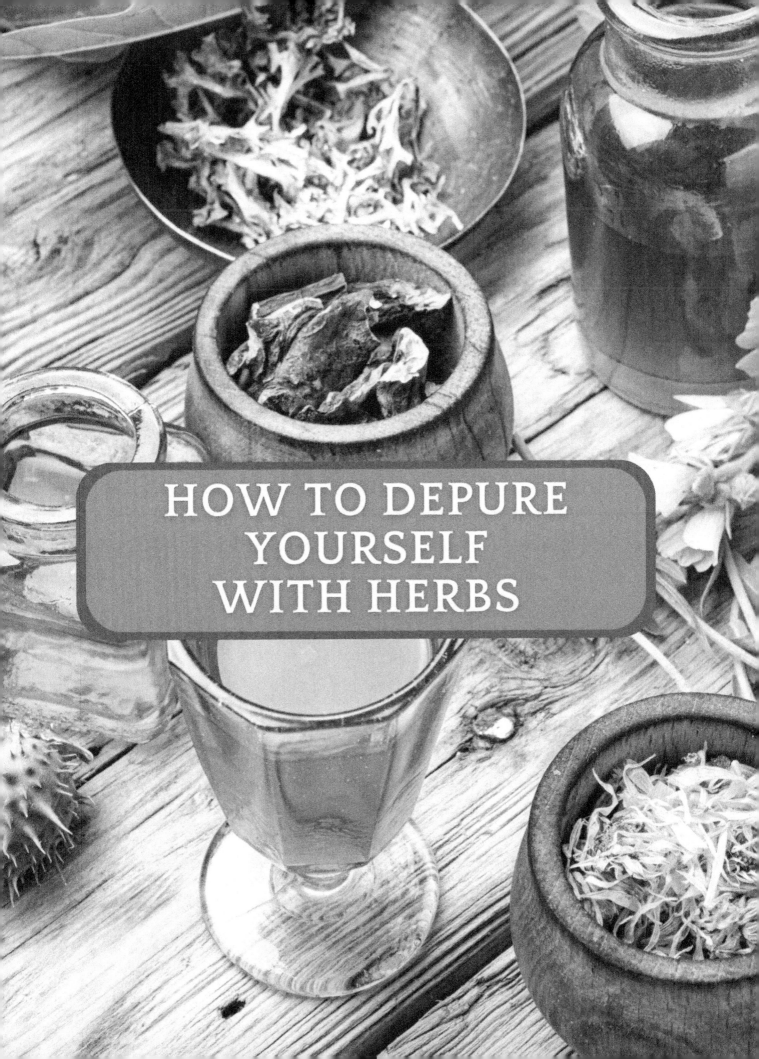

HOW TO DEPURE YOURSELF WITH HERBS

Chapter 1

DETOX AND PURIFICATION IMPORTANCE

Detox and purification have become popular terms in recent years, with many people looking for ways to cleanse their bodies and improve their overall health.

Detoxification involves removing toxins from the body, while purification aims to improve overall health and wellbeing through the use of natural methods. Both detox and purification are important for maintaining optimal health, and can be achieved through a combination of diet, exercise, and other lifestyle changes. The human body is constantly exposed to toxins from a variety of sources, including pollution, pesticides, processed foods, and stress. These toxins can accumulate in the body over time and lead to a range of health problems, including fatigue, headaches, allergies, and digestive issues. Detoxification is the process of removing these toxins from the body, allowing the body to function more efficiently and reducing the risk of disease.

There are several ways to detoxify the body, including fasting, juicing, and using herbs and supplements. Fasting involves abstaining from food for a period of time, allowing the body to focus its energy on detoxification. Juicing involves consuming fresh fruit and vegetable juices, which are rich in antioxidants and other nutrients that support detoxification. Herbs and supplements can also be used to support the body's natural detoxification processes, such as milk thistle, dandelion root, and turmeric.

Purification is a broader term that encompasses not only the removal of toxins from the body, but also the promotion of overall health and wellbeing. This can be achieved through a combination of diet, exercise, and other lifestyle changes. Eating a diet rich in whole, unprocessed foods, and avoiding processed and sugary foods can help to support the body's natural purification processes. Regular exercise, stress reduction techniques, and getting enough sleep are also important for maintaining optimal health and promoting purification. Detoxification and purification can also have a positive impact on mental and emotional wellbeing. By removing toxins from the body and promoting overall health and wellbeing, individuals may experience increased energy, improved mood, and greater clarity of thought. This can lead to improved productivity, better relationships, and an overall better quality of life.

While detoxification and purification are important for maintaining optimal health, it is important to approach these practices with caution. Extreme fasting or detox programs can be harmful and should only be undertaken under the supervision of a qualified healthcare practitioner. Detoxification and purification are important for maintaining optimal health and wellbeing. By removing toxins from the body and promoting overall health and wellbeing, individuals can experience increased energy, improved mood, and greater clarity of thought.

WHAT DOES IT MEAN TO DETOX

Detox, short for detoxification, is a process that helps eliminate harmful toxins from the body. Our bodies have a natural detoxification system that works to keep us healthy, but sometimes it can become overloaded due to poor diet, environmental toxins, stress, and other factors. When this happens, it can be beneficial to give the body a helping hand by implementing a detoxification protocol.

Detoxification is a holistic approach to health that focuses on cleansing the body of toxins and restoring balance to the body's natural processes. It involves not only the physical body but also the mind and emotions. By removing harmful substances from the body, we can improve our overall health and well-being, reduce the risk of disease, and improve the function of our organs.

Toxins are everywhere. They are in the air we breathe, the water we drink, the food we eat, and the products we use. Over time, these toxins can accumulate in the body and lead to a range of health problems, including chronic fatigue, allergies, headaches, skin conditions, digestive issues, and more. By detoxifying the body, we can remove these harmful substances and give our bodies the chance to heal and regenerate.

Detoxification is also important for weight loss. When the body is overloaded with toxins, it can be difficult to lose weight, even with proper diet and exercise. By removing these toxins, the body can more easily burn fat and shed excess weight.

In addition, detoxification can improve mental clarity, boost energy levels, and enhance the immune system. It can also help reduce inflammation in the body, which is a common factor in many chronic diseases. Detoxification is not a one-time event but rather an ongoing process. Adopting healthy habits such as a balanced diet, regular exercise, and proper hydration can help support the body's natural detoxification system and promote optimal health. Detoxification is a powerful tool for improving health and well-being. By removing harmful toxins from the body, we can reduce the risk of disease, enhance our energy and vitality, and improve mental clarity. There are many different approaches to detoxification, and it is important to find a method that works for you. By making detoxification a regular part of your wellness routine, you can help your body function at its best and enjoy optimal health for years to come.

HOW TO DETOX AND STAY FIT

Detoxing refers to the process of eliminating toxins and waste products from the body. The body has its own detoxification system, which involves the liver, kidneys, skin, and lungs. However, due to poor diet, exposure to environmental toxins, stress, and other factors, the body's natural detoxification process can become overwhelmed, leading to a buildup of toxins and waste products in the body. This can contribute to a variety of health problems, including fatigue, poor digestion, skin problems, and more.

Fortunately, there are several ways to support the body's natural detoxification process and promote overall health and fitness. Here are some tips on how to detox and stay fit:

- **Eat a Healthy Diet:** A healthy diet is essential for supporting the body's natural detoxification process. This means eating plenty of fruits, vegetables, whole grains, lean proteins, and healthy fats. Avoid processed foods, sugary drinks, and other unhealthy foods that can contribute to inflammation and disrupt the body's natural detoxification process.

- **Stay Hydrated:** Drinking plenty of water is essential for flushing toxins out of the body. Aim to drink at least 8-10 glasses of water per day, and consider adding lemon or lime to your water to boost detoxification.

- **Exercise Regularly:** Regular exercise is essential for promoting overall health and fitness. Exercise helps to boost circulation, support the lymphatic system, and promote the elimination of toxins from the body. Aim for at least 30 minutes of moderate exercise per day, such as walking, jogging, cycling, or yoga.

- **Practice Stress-Reduction Techniques:** Chronic stress can disrupt the body's natural detoxification process and contribute to a variety of health problems. To support detoxification and overall health, it's important to practice stress-reduction techniques such as meditation, deep breathing, yoga, or massage.

- **Try Detoxifying Foods and Supplements:** There are several foods and supplements that can support the body's natural detoxification process. These include foods like beets, broccoli, garlic, and ginger, as well as supplements like milk thistle, dandelion root, and N-acetyl cysteine.

- **Get Plenty of Sleep:** Sleep is essential for overall health and wellbeing, and it's also important for supporting the body's natural detoxification process. Aim for at least 7-8 hours of sleep per night, and consider practicing relaxation techniques before bed to help promote restful sleep

- **Avoid Toxins:** To support detoxification, it's important to avoid exposure to toxins as much as possible. This means avoiding tobacco smoke, alcohol, and other drugs, as well as reducing exposure to environmental toxins such as air pollution, pesticides, and other chemicals.

REACTIVATE YOUR MUSCLE TONE

Muscle tone refers to the natural tension or firmness of your muscles at rest. Over time, muscle tone can decrease due to inactivity or aging. However, it's possible to reactivate and improve muscle tone through regular exercise and a healthy lifestyle. In this article, we'll discuss some tips on how to reactivate your muscle tone.

- **Start with a Warm-up:** Before any workout, it's important to warm up your muscles. A warm-up will help to prepare your muscles for exercise, prevent injury, and increase blood flow. A good warm-up should include light cardio such as jogging or jumping jacks, followed by dynamic stretches such as lunges, arm circles, and leg swings.

- **Resistance Training:** Resistance training is an effective way to reactivate muscle tone. It involves working against a resistance, such as weight lifting or using resistance bands. Resistance training helps to build and strengthen muscles, improve bone density, and increase metabolism. It's recommended to do resistance training at least two to three times per week.

- **Cardiovascular Exercise:** Cardiovascular exercise, also known as aerobic exercise, is important for overall fitness and health. It can also help to reactivate muscle tone by burning fat and increasing muscle definition. Some examples of cardiovascular exercise include running, cycling, swimming, and dancing. It's recommended to do cardiovascular exercise at least three to five times per week for at least 30 minutes per session.

- **Yoga and Pilates:** Yoga and Pilates are both low-impact forms of exercise that can help to reactivate muscle tone. They focus on building strength, flexibility, and balance. Yoga and Pilates can also help to improve posture and reduce stress. It's recommended to do yoga or Pilates at least once or twice per week.

- **Stay Hydrated and Eat a Healthy Diet:** Drinking enough water and eating a healthy diet are important for muscle health and overall fitness. Staying hydrated helps to flush out toxins and prevent muscle cramps. Eating a balanced diet that includes lean protein, complex carbohydrates, and healthy fats provides your body with the nutrients it needs to build and repair muscles.

- **Get Enough Rest and Recovery:** Rest and recovery are essential for muscle growth and reactivation. It's important to give your muscles time to recover between workouts. This means taking rest days and getting enough sleep. Aim for seven to eight hours of sleep per night to help your muscles recover and reactivate.

Chapter 2

PURIFYING RECIPES

KIDNEYS

1. Fennel and Milk Thistle Herbal Tea

Ingredients:

- 1 tablespoon of fennel seeds

- 1 tablespoon of milk thistle seeds

- 2 cups of filtered water

- Honey or lemon juice (optional)

Instructions:

- Add fennel seeds and milk thistle seeds to a teapot or heat-resistant glass container.

- Pour 2 cups of filtered water over the seeds and let it steep for 15-20 minutes.

- Strain the tea using a fine-mesh strainer or cheesecloth.

- Add honey or lemon juice to taste (optional).

- Serve hot or cold.

Note: Fennel and milk thistle are two herbs that are traditionally known for their beneficial effects on kidney function. Fennel contains antioxidants and diuretic properties that help to flush out toxins and excess fluids from the body, including the kidneys. Milk thistle has been found to support liver and kidney health by promoting the regeneration of damaged cells.

This herbal tea can be consumed regularly as part of a kidney cleanse or as a preventative measure to maintain healthy kidney function. It is important to note that if you have any underlying medical conditions or are taking medications, it is best to consult with your healthcare provider before adding this tea to your routine.

Enjoy this delicious and purifying herbal tea as a refreshing and healthy addition to your daily routine.

2. Fennel and Artichoke Infusion

Ingredients:

- 1 large artichoke, chopped into small pieces

- 1 tablespoon of fennel seeds

- 4 cups of water

- Honey (optional)

Instructions:

- Bring 4 cups of water to a boil in a pot.

- Add the chopped artichoke and fennel seeds to the pot.

- Reduce the heat to low and let the mixture simmer for 10-15 minutes.

- After 15 minutes, remove the pot from heat and let it cool down.

- Strain the mixture using a fine mesh strainer into a pitcher.

- Add honey to taste (optional).

- Serve the infusion warm or cold.

Note: This infusion is a great way to support your kidney health. Both fennel and artichoke are known for their detoxifying and diuretic properties, which can help flush out toxins and excess fluids from the body. Additionally, artichoke is a good source of antioxidants and can help regulate cholesterol levels. It's important to note that if you have any pre-existing medical conditions or are taking medications, you should consult with your healthcare provider before adding any new herbal remedies to your routine.

3. Lentil and Turmeric Soup

Ingredients:

- 2 cups of lentils, rinsed and drained

- 6 cups of water

- 1 tablespoon of olive oil

- 1 onion, chopped

- 4 cloves of garlic, minced

- 1 tablespoon of grated ginger

- 2 tsps of ground turmeric

- 1 tsp of cumin

- 1 tsp of paprika

- 1/2 tsp of black pepper

- 2 carrots, chopped

- 2 celery stalks, chopped

- 1 red bell pepper, chopped

- 4 cups of vegetable broth

- Salt to taste

Instructions:

- Heat the olive oil in a large pot over medium heat. Add the onion, garlic, and ginger, and sauté until the onion is translucent, about 5 minutes.

- Add the turmeric, cumin, paprika, and black pepper, and sauté for another minute.

- Add the lentils, carrots, celery, red bell pepper, water, and vegetable broth to the pot. Stir to combine.

- Bring the mixture to a boil, then reduce the heat and simmer for about 30 minutes or until the lentils are soft and fully cooked.

- Remove the pot from the heat and let the soup cool slightly.

- Using an immersion blender or regular blender, puree the soup until smooth.

- Season with salt to taste.

- Serve the soup hot, garnished with fresh herbs if desired.

Note: Lentil and turmeric soup is a delicious and nutritious dish that is perfect for promoting kidney health. Lentils are a great source of protein and fiber, while turmeric is a powerful anti-inflammatory spice that has been shown to have beneficial effects on kidney function.

4. Mint and Licorice Infusion

Ingredients:

- 1 tablespoon of dried mint leaves

- 1 tablespoon of dried licorice root

- 4 cups of filtered water

- Honey or lemon (optional)

Instructions:

- In a medium-sized pot, bring the filtered water to a boil.

- Once the water is boiling, add in the dried mint leaves and licorice root.

- Reduce the heat to low and let the herbs steep in the water for 10-15 minutes.

- After 10-15 minutes, remove the pot from the heat and strain the infusion using a fine mesh strainer.

- If desired, add a tsp of honey or a squeeze of lemon for taste.

- Serve hot or cold.

Note: Mint and licorice are both known for their potential health benefits for the kidneys. Mint is believed to have diuretic properties, which can help the kidneys flush out toxins and excess fluids. Licorice root is said to have anti-inflammatory properties and may help protect the kidneys from damage caused by inflammation. This refreshing and soothing infusion can be enjoyed any time of the day as part of a healthy and kidney-friendly diet.

I want you to write a unique recipe content in the right format on Gramigna and dandelion herbal tea for kidney

5. Gramigna and Dandelion Herbal Tea

Ingredients:

- 1 tablespoon dried Gramigna (also known as Agropyron repens)

- 1 tablespoon dried Dandelion root

- 2 cups water

- Lemon juice and honey (optional)

Instructions:

- Boil 2 cups of water in a saucepan.

- Add the dried Gramigna and Dandelion root to the boiling water.

- Lower the heat and let the herbs simmer for 10-15 minutes.

- Remove the saucepan from heat and let it cool down for a few minutes.

- Strain the tea into a cup.

- If you prefer, add a squeeze of fresh lemon juice and a drizzle of honey for added flavor and benefits.

- Enjoy your Gramigna and Dandelion Herbal Tea.

Note: Gramigna and Dandelion Herbal Tea is known for its detoxifying properties that help to support kidney health. Gramigna is a diuretic herb that helps to increase urine output, which in turn helps to flush out toxins from the kidneys. Dandelion root is a natural diuretic and also has anti-inflammatory properties that help to reduce inflammation in the kidneys.

LIVER

1. Cumin and Rosemary Herbal Tea

Ingredients:

- 2 tsps cumin seeds

- 1 tsp dried rosemary leaves

- 4 cups of water

- Honey or lemon juice (optional)

Instructions:

- In a small pan, dry roast cumin seeds on low heat for 2-3 minutes or until fragrant.

- Crush the roasted cumin seeds using a mortar and pestle or a spice grinder.

- Add crushed cumin seeds and dried rosemary leaves to a tea infuser or a tea bag.

- In a medium saucepan, bring 4 cups of water to a boil.

- Turn off the heat and add the tea infuser or tea bag to the water.

- Cover and let the herbs steep for 5-10 minutes.

- Remove the tea infuser or tea bag and discard.

- Pour the tea into a cup and add honey or lemon juice if desired.

Note: Cumin and rosemary are both known for their ability to support liver function. Cumin helps stimulate the production of digestive enzymes and aids in the digestion of fats, while rosemary contains antioxidants that protect the liver from damage. Drinking this herbal tea regularly can help support a healthy liver.

2. Carrot and Fennel Infusion

Ingredients:

- 2 large carrots, sliced

- 1 fennel bulb, sliced

- 4 cups of water

- 1 tbsp honey

- 1 tsp lemon juice

- Fresh mint leaves for garnish

Instructions:

- In a large pot, bring 4 cups of water to a boil.

- Add the sliced carrots and fennel to the pot and let it boil for 5-7 minutes.

- Reduce the heat and let the mixture simmer for another 10 minutes.

- Remove from heat and let it cool down for a few minutes.

- Strain the mixture and pour the liquid into a large bowl or pitcher.

- Add honey and lemon juice and stir well.

- Serve the infusion warm and garnish with fresh mint leaves.

Note: Carrots are rich in beta-carotene and other antioxidants that help to detoxify the liver. Fennel is also rich in antioxidants and has anti-inflammatory properties that aid in liver function. Honey and lemon juice add natural sweetness and tanginess to the infusion, making it a delicious and healthy beverage option. This infusion can be consumed daily, preferably in the morning or after a meal. Enjoy the benefits of this natural liver detoxifier and feel refreshed and rejuvenated.

3. SAVORY BROTH with CABBAGE and OLIVE OIL

Ingredients:

- 1 head of cabbage, chopped

- 1 large onion, diced

- 4 garlic cloves, minced

- 2 tablespoons of olive oil

- 1 tsp of dried thyme

- 1 tsp of dried sage

- 6 cups of vegetable broth

- Salt and pepper to taste

Instructions:

- In a large pot, heat the olive oil over medium heat. Add the onion and garlic and sauté until translucent, about 5 minutes.

- Add the chopped cabbage and stir until coated with the oil and onion mixture.

- Add the dried thyme and sage to the pot and stir.

- Pour in the vegetable broth and stir to combine. Bring the broth to a boil, then reduce the heat to low and let simmer for 30 minutes.

- After 30 minutes, remove the pot from the heat and let cool for a few minutes.

- Using an immersion blender or regular blender, puree the soup until smooth.

- Season with salt and pepper to taste.

- Serve hot, garnished with a drizzle of olive oil.

Note: This savory broth with cabbage and olive oil is a delicious and healthy recipe that is specifically designed to support liver health. Cabbage is rich in antioxidants and helps to improve liver function, while olive oil contains healthy fats that are beneficial for the liver. This recipe is also vegan and gluten-free, making it a great option for people with dietary restrictions. Enjoy this flavorful broth as a starter or main dish, and feel good knowing that you're giving your liver the nutrients it needs to stay healthy.

4. Beetroot and Chicory Infusion

Ingredients:

- 1 medium beetroot, peeled and chopped

- 1 head of chicory, chopped

- 4 cups of water

- Juice of 1/2 a lemon

- 1 tablespoon of honey (optional)

Instructions:

- In a large pot, bring 4 cups of water to a boil.

- Add the chopped beetroot and chicory to the pot.

- Reduce the heat to medium-low and let the mixture simmer for 10-15 minutes.

- Remove the pot from heat and strain the infusion into a bowl, using a fine mesh strainer to remove any solids.

- Allow the infusion to cool for a few minutes, then stir in the lemon juice and honey (if using).

- Serve the infusion warm or chilled, depending on your preference.

Note: Beetroot and Chicory Infusion is packed with antioxidants and nutrients that are great for supporting liver health. The beetroot contains betaine, which helps protect the liver from damage, while chicory is rich in compounds that stimulate bile production and aid in digestion. The lemon juice adds a refreshing zing to the infusion, while the honey provides a touch of sweetness to balance out the bitterness of the chicory. Enjoy!

5. Lemon and Grapefruit Herbal Tea

Ingredients:

- 1 lemon

- 1 grapefruit

- 1 tablespoon of honey

- 2 cups of water

- 2 sprigs of fresh mint

Instructions:

- Cut the lemon and grapefruit into thin slices.

- In a pot, add the sliced lemon and grapefruit to 2 cups of water.

- Bring the mixture to a boil and let it simmer for 10-15 minutes.

- Remove from heat and add the honey, stirring until it dissolves.

- Let the mixture cool for a few minutes.

- Add the fresh mint sprigs and let it steep for 5-10 minutes.

- Strain the tea to remove any solids.

- Serve hot or cold.

Note: This herbal tea is rich in antioxidants and vitamin C, which are both beneficial for liver health. The grapefruit contains naringenin, which has been shown to help protect the liver from damage. The lemon and honey also aid in digestion and promote overall liver function. The addition of fresh mint gives this tea a refreshing taste and can help to soothe an upset stomach. Enjoy this delicious and healthy tea as part of your liver detox routine.

DIABETES

1. Apple and Melon Infusion

Ingredients:

- 1 medium-sized apple, sliced

- 1/2 small cantaloupe melon, diced

- 4 cups of water

- 1 cinnamon stick

- 1 tsp of honey (optional)

- Ice cubes

Instructions:

- Rinse the apple and cantaloupe melon in cold water, then slice and dice them respectively.

- In a medium-sized saucepan, add water and cinnamon stick, and bring to a boil.

- Once boiling, add the sliced apple and diced cantaloupe melon to the saucepan.

- Reduce the heat and let it simmer for 10-15 minutes, stirring occasionally.

- Remove the saucepan from heat and let it cool for 5 minutes.

- Strain the mixture using a fine mesh sieve or cheesecloth, into a pitcher.

- Add honey to sweeten (optional).

- Chill in the refrigerator for at least 2 hours.

- Before serving, add ice cubes and garnish with a slice of apple or cantaloupe melon.

Note: This Apple and Melon Infusion is a refreshing and healthy beverage that can be enjoyed as a delicious and natural way to hydrate your body. It is also ideal for people with diabetes as it is low in sugar and high in vitamins and minerals. The combination of apple and cantaloupe melon provides a good source of fiber, vitamin C, and antioxidants, which can help improve digestion and boost the immune system. Enjoy this infusion any time of the day for a delicious and healthy beverage.

2. Raspberry and Lemon Herbal Tea

Ingredients:

- 1/2 cup fresh raspberries

- 2-3 slices of fresh lemon

- 1 tsp honey (optional)

- 2 cups water

- 1-2 tea bags of raspberry herbal tea (optional)

Instructions:

- Rinse the raspberries and lemon slices with cold water.

- In a small pot, bring 2 cups of water to a boil.

- Add the raspberries and lemon slices to the pot of boiling water and let it simmer for 10-15 minutes.

- Remove the pot from heat and let it cool down for a couple of minutes.

- Strain the mixture into a cup or teapot, discarding the solids.

- If desired, add a tsp of honey to sweeten.

- If desired, add 1-2 tea bags of raspberry herbal tea to enhance the flavor.

- Stir well and serve hot.

Note: This herbal tea is rich in antioxidants and vitamin C from the raspberries and lemon, which help to boost the immune system and promote healthy skin. The tea is also low in sugar and calories, making it a great option for those with diabetes or watching their calorie intake.

3. Chickpea, Garlic, and Sage Soup

Ingredients:

- 2 cans of chickpeas, drained and rinsed

- 1 onion, diced

- 4 garlic cloves, minced

- 4 cups of low-sodium chicken or vegetable broth

- 1 tsp of dried sage

- 1 tsp of ground cumin

- Salt and pepper to taste

- 1 tablespoon of olive oil

Instructions:

- Heat olive oil in a large pot over medium-high heat.

- Add onion and garlic, sauté until onion is soft and translucent.

- Add the chickpeas, sage, cumin, salt, and pepper to the pot.

- Stir the ingredients well and cook for 2-3 minutes.

- Add the broth and bring the mixture to a boil.

- Reduce the heat and let it simmer for 15-20 minutes until the chickpeas are tender and the soup has thickened.

- Remove from heat and let it cool for a few minutes.

- Blend the soup using an immersion blender or transfer the soup to a blender and blend until smooth.

- Return the soup to the pot and reheat over low heat until it is heated through.

Note: This soup is high in fiber and protein from the chickpeas, which can help regulate blood sugar levels in those with diabetes. The garlic and sage add a depth of flavor while also providing antioxidant and anti-inflammatory benefits. It's a delicious and nutritious option for a diabetes-friendly meal.

4. Strawberry and Cinnamon Herbal Tea

Ingredients:

- 1 cup fresh strawberries, sliced

- 2 cinnamon sticks

- 4 cups water

Instructions:

- Rinse the fresh strawberries and slice them into small pieces.

- In a pot, add the sliced strawberries and cinnamon sticks with 4 cups of water and bring to a boil.

- Reduce the heat and let the mixture simmer for 10 minutes.

- Remove the pot from heat and let it cool down to room temperature.

- Strain the liquid to remove the strawberry and cinnamon bits.

- Pour the tea into a mug and enjoy.

- You can add a tsp of honey for sweetness if desired.

- Serve this tea chilled for a refreshing summer beverage.

Note: Strawberries and cinnamon both have natural anti-inflammatory properties and may help to regulate blood sugar levels. This Strawberry and Cinnamon Herbal Tea is a delicious and refreshing way to manage blood sugar levels for those with diabetes. This tea can be enjoyed any time of the day and can be served hot or cold, making it a versatile beverage option. The natural anti-inflammatory properties of strawberries and cinnamon make it a healthy addition to any diet

5. Ginger and Lime Infusion for Diabetes

Ingredients:

- 1 lime, sliced

- 2-inch piece of ginger root, sliced

- 4 cups of water

- Honey (optional)

Instructions:

- In a medium saucepan, add the sliced lime and ginger root.

- Pour in the water and bring to a boil.

- Once boiling, reduce heat and let it simmer for 10-15 minutes.

- Strain the mixture and discard the lime and ginger pieces.

- If desired, add honey to taste.

- Pour the ginger and lime infusion into mugs and enjoy.

Note: Ginger and lime both have anti-inflammatory properties, which can help regulate blood sugar levels in people with diabetes. Ginger also contains compounds that may improve insulin sensitivity, while lime is a good source of vitamin C, an antioxidant that can help reduce the risk of complications associated with diabetes. This infusion is a delicious and healthy alternative to sugary drinks, making it a great choice for those looking to manage their blood sugar levels naturally.

HYPERTENSION

1. Pomegranate and Red Fruit Infusion

Ingredients:

- 1/2 cup pomegranate seeds

- 1/2 cup mixed red fruits (such as raspberries, strawberries, and cherries)

- 2 cinnamon sticks

- 4 cups water

Instructions:

- Rinse the pomegranate seeds and mixed red fruits in cold water and set aside.

- In a medium-sized saucepan, bring 4 cups of water to a boil over medium-high heat.

- Add the cinnamon sticks and reduce the heat to low. Let the cinnamon sticks simmer for 5 minutes.

- Add the pomegranate seeds and mixed red fruits to the saucepan and let them simmer for an additional 5-10 minutes, until the fruits are soft and the water has turned a deep red color.

- Remove the saucepan from the heat and let the mixture cool for 5 minutes.

- Strain the mixture through a fine-mesh strainer or cheesecloth, discarding the solids.

- Serve the pomegranate and red fruit infusion hot or chilled, with a cinnamon stick as a garnish if desired.

Note: This infusion is packed with antioxidants from the pomegranate seeds and mixed red fruits, and the cinnamon adds a subtle spice that can help improve blood circulation. It is a great way to stay hydrated while also helping to regulate blood pressure. Enjoy!

2. Coriander and Cardamom Herbal Tea

Ingredients:

- 2 tablespoons coriander seeds

- 1 tsp cardamom pods

- 4 cups water

Instructions:

- Crush the coriander seeds and cardamom pods with a mortar and pestle to release their oils.

- Boil the water in a pot and add the crushed coriander seeds and cardamom pods.

- Reduce heat and let the mixture simmer for 10-15 minutes.

- Strain the tea through a fine-mesh strainer into a teapot or individual mugs.

- Serve hot and enjoy!

Note: Coriander and cardamom are both known for their blood pressure-lowering effects. This herbal tea can be a great addition to a healthy diet and lifestyle to manage hypertension. However, it is important to consult with a healthcare professional before making any significant changes to your diet or treatment plan.

3. Broth of Beans, Celery, and Cumin

Ingredients:

- 1 cup of white beans

- 3 cups of water

- 2 celery stalks, chopped

- 1 onion, chopped

- 1 garlic clove, minced

- 2 tablespoons of olive oil

- 1 tsp of cumin

- Salt and pepper to taste

Instructions:

- Soak the white beans in water overnight.

- Drain the beans and rinse them under cold water. In a large pot, heat the olive oil over medium heat.

- Add the chopped onion and celery and sauté until softened, for about 5 minutes.

- Add the minced garlic and cook for another minute.

- Add the drained beans to the pot and stir to combine.

- Add the water and bring to a boil.

- Reduce the heat to low, cover the pot and let it simmer for about an hour or until the beans are tender.

- Once the beans are cooked, remove the pot from the heat and let it cool for a few minutes.

- Using an immersion blender, blend the soup until smooth.

- Add the cumin and season with salt and pepper to taste.

- Serve hot and enjoy!

Note: This delicious and healthy Broth of Beans, Celery, and Cumin is a great option for people with hypertension who want to incorporate more heart-healthy foods into their diet.

4. Infusion of Celery and Cucumber

Ingredients:

- 1 medium-sized cucumber, sliced

- 2 stalks of celery, chopped

- 4 cups of water

- 1 tsp of honey (optional)

Instructions:

- Bring the water to a boil in a medium-sized pot.

- Add the sliced cucumber and chopped celery to the boiling water.

- Reduce heat to low and let the mixture simmer for about 10-15 minutes.

- Turn off the heat and let the infusion cool down for a few minutes.

- Strain the infusion to remove the cucumber and celery pieces.

- If desired, add honey to sweeten the infusion.

- Serve hot or cold.

Note: Both celery and cucumber have natural diuretic properties, which can help lower blood pressure by reducing the volume of fluid in the body. Additionally, this infusion is low in sodium and high in potassium, which can also help regulate blood pressure. It's important to note that while natural remedies like this can be beneficial, they should not be used as a substitute for medical treatment. If you have hypertension or any other health concerns, be sure to consult with your healthcare provider.

5. Cardamom and Saffron Herbal Tea

Ingredients:

- 4 cups of water

- 4-5 cardamom pods

- 1/4 tsp saffron threads

- Honey or any other sweetener, to taste

Instructions:

- In a saucepan, bring 4 cups of water to a boil.

- Once the water has boiled, add 4-5 cardamom pods and 1/4 tsp of saffron threads to the water.

- Reduce the heat and let the mixture simmer for 5-10 minutes.

- After simmering, remove the saucepan from heat and let the tea cool for a few minutes.

- Strain the tea into a cup or teapot.

- Add honey or any other sweetener of your choice, to taste.

- Serve hot and enjoy!

Note: Both cardamom and saffron have anti-inflammatory properties, which can be beneficial for reducing high blood pressure. This tea is not only healthy but also has a delicious, fragrant taste that you'll love.

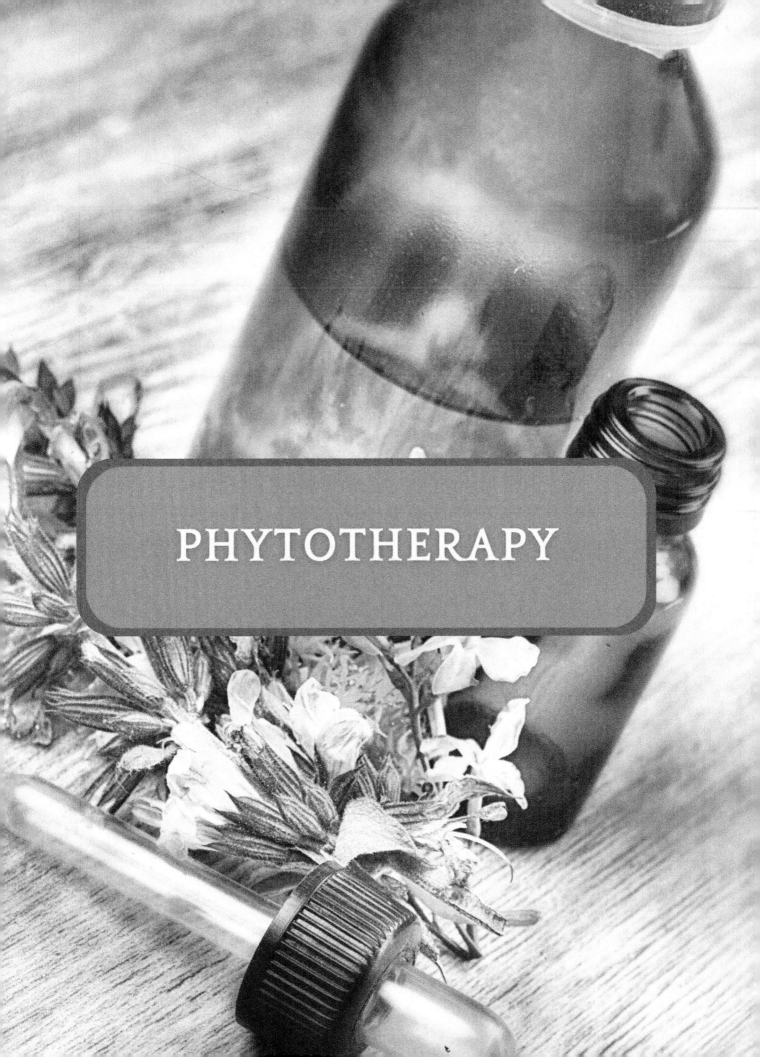

PHYTOTHERAPY

Chapter 1

WHAT IS PHYTOTHERAPY?

Phytotherapy is the use of plants or their derivatives for therapeutic purposes. It is an ancient practice that has been used for thousands of years to treat various illnesses and promote overall health and well-being. In recent years, phytotherapy has gained popularity as a natural alternative to conventional medicine, particularly for those who seek to avoid the side effects associated with pharmaceutical drugs.

Phytotherapy is based on the belief that plants contain active compounds that have medicinal properties. These compounds can be extracted from the plant and used to treat a variety of conditions. For example, the active ingredient in aspirin, salicylic acid, was originally derived from the bark of the willow tree.

There are many different types of plants used in phytotherapy, and each plant contains a unique combination of active compounds. Some of the most commonly used plants in phytotherapy include echinacea, ginkgo biloba, St. John's wort, and chamomile. Echinacea is a popular herb used to boost the immune system and prevent infections. It is often used to treat colds, flu, and other respiratory infections. Echinacea is available in various forms, including capsules, tinctures, and teas. Ginkgo biloba is an herb commonly used to improve cognitive function and memory. It is believed to work by increasing blood flow to the brain and protecting the brain from oxidative stress. Ginkgo biloba is available in various forms, including capsules, tablets, and teas. St. John's wort is an herb commonly used to treat mild to moderate depression. It is believed to work by increasing levels of serotonin in the brain. St. John's wort is available in various forms, including capsules, tablets, and teas. Chamomile is an herb commonly used to promote relaxation and reduce anxiety. It is often used as a sleep aid and is believed to work by promoting the production of GABA, a neurotransmitter that helps to calm the brain. Chamomile is available in various forms, including teas, tinctures, and essential oils.

Phytotherapy can be used to treat a wide range of conditions, from minor ailments such as headaches and colds to more serious conditions such as cancer and heart disease. It can be used alone or in combination with conventional medicine, depending on the individual's needs and preferences. One of the advantages of phytotherapy is that it is generally considered to be safe when used as directed. However, like any other form of treatment, it is important to use caution and consult a healthcare provider before beginning any new herbal regimen, especially if you are taking prescription medications or have a pre-existing medical condition.

In conclusion, phytotherapy is a natural and effective way to promote health and well- being. It has been used for thousands of years to treat a variety of conditions and is gaining popularity as a natural alternative to conventional medicine. By using plants and their derivatives, phytotherapy offers a safe and effective way to maintain optimal health and wellness.

PHISTORY AND EVOLUTION OF PHYTOTHERAPY

hytotherapy, also known as herbal medicine or botanical medicine, is the practice of using plants and plant extracts for medicinal purposes. It is one of the oldest forms of medicine and has been practiced for centuries across cultures around the world.

The history of phytotherapy can be traced back to ancient civilizations like the Egyptians, Greeks, and Romans, who used plant extracts for healing and treating various ailments.

In ancient Egypt, medicinal plants were used extensively for treating a wide range of health problems. The Ebbers Papyrus, which dates back to 1550 BC, is an ancient Egyptian medical text that contains detailed descriptions of over 800 plant-based remedies. Many of these remedies are still used today in modern phytotherapy. The Greeks and Romans also used plants for medicinal purposes. Hippocrates, the father of modern medicine, advocated for the use of plants as medicine and wrote extensively on the subject. The Roman physician Galen also wrote about the medicinal properties of plants, and his works influenced the development of medicine in Europe for centuries.

During the Middle Ages, phytotherapy was practiced extensively in Europe. Monks and herbalists grew and studied plants for medicinal purposes, and their knowledge was passed down through generations.

In the 16th century, the Swiss physician Paracelsus further developed the use of plants for medicinal purposes and introduced the concept of using specific parts of plants for specific ailments.

In the 19th century, the development of modern medicine led to a decline in the use of phytotherapy. Synthetic drugs became popular, and many medical practitioners turned away from traditional plant-based remedies. However, in the mid-20th century, there was a renewed interest in phytotherapy, particularly in Europe, where it is still widely used today.

In the 21st century, phytotherapy has become increasingly popular worldwide. With a growing interest in natural and holistic approaches to healthcare, many people are turning to plant-based remedies for various ailments. Phytotherapy is now recognized as an important field of study and research, with many universities offering programs in herbal medicine and pharmacognosy (the study of natural product drugs). The evolution of phytotherapy has also been shaped by advancements in technology and science. Today, modern scientific methods are used to study the active compounds in plants and understand their medicinal properties. This has led to the development of standardized herbal extracts and supplements, which are widely available in health food stores and pharmacies.

The history of phytotherapy is rich and diverse, spanning many centuries and cultures. From ancient Egypt to modern times, the use of plants for medicinal purposes has been an important part of human healthcare. While there have been periods of decline, the renewed interest in natural and holistic approaches to healthcare has led to a resurgence of interest in phytotherapy. With ongoing research and advancements in technology, the future of phytotherapy looks bright, with the potential to provide safe and effective remedies for a wide range of health problems.

IMPORTANCE OF PHYTOTHERAPY

Phytotherapy, also known as herbal medicine, is the use of plants or plant extracts for medicinal purposes. It has been used for thousands of years and is still an important part of healthcare in many parts of the world. Here are some of the key reasons why phytotherapy is important:

NATURAL AND SUSTAINABLE: One of the main advantages of phytotherapy is that it is a natural and sustainable form of medicine. Unlike synthetic drugs, which are often made from non-renewable resources and can have harmful side effects, herbal remedies are made from plants that can be grown and harvested sustainably. This makes phytotherapy a more environmentally friendly choice.

WIDE RANGE OF APPLICATIONS: Herbal remedies can be used to treat a wide range of health conditions, from minor ailments like headaches and digestive problems to more serious conditions like cancer and heart disease. This versatility is due to the fact that plants contain a vast array of chemical compounds that can have beneficial effects on the body.

ACCESSIBLE AND AFFORDABLE: Phytotherapy is often more accessible and affordable than conventional medicine, particularly in developing countries where modern healthcare systems may be lacking. Many herbal remedies can be grown in a backyard garden or collected from the wild, making them readily available to people who may not have access to modern medical facilities.

PERSONALIZED TREATMENT: Herbal remedies can be tailored to the individual, taking into account factors such as age, gender, and overall health. This personalized approach can lead to better outcomes and fewer side effects compared to one-size-fits-all treatments.

PREVENTION OF CHRONIC DISEASES: Herbal remedies can be used to prevent chronic diseases such as diabetes, heart disease, and cancer. This is because many plants contain antioxidant and anti-inflammatory compounds that can protect the body against damage from free radicals and inflammation, two processes that are believed to contribute to the development of chronic diseases.

COMPLEMENTARY TO CONVENTIONAL MEDICINE: Phytotherapy can also be used in combination with conventional medicine to enhance its effectiveness or reduce side effects. For example, some herbal remedies can help to reduce nausea and vomiting caused by chemotherapy, or improve the absorption of certain drugs.

In conclusion, phytotherapy is a natural, versatile, and sustainable form of medicine that has many important benefits. It can be used to treat a wide range of health conditions, is accessible and affordable, can be tailored to the individual, and can even help to prevent chronic diseases. While it is not a panacea, it is an important tool in the healthcare toolkit and is likely to continue to play a role in healthcare for many years to come.

Chapter 2

PHYTOTHERAPY RECIPES

Seasonal Evils

I. FEVER: LAUREL AND LEMON BALM HERBAL TEA

Ingredients:

- 1 tablespoon dried laurel leaves

- 2 tablespoons dried lemon balm leaves

- 4 cups water

- Honey (optional)

Instructions:

- Bring 4 cups of water to a boil in a medium saucepan.

- Add the dried laurel leaves and lemon balm leaves to the boiling water.

- Reduce the heat to low and let the tea simmer for 10-15 minutes.

- Remove the saucepan from the heat and let the tea cool for a few minutes.

- Strain the tea using a fine mesh strainer or cheesecloth.

- Serve the tea hot and add honey to taste, if desired.

Note: Laurel leaves have antibacterial and antiviral properties, and are known to help reduce fever. Lemon balm is also antiviral and is known to have calming and soothing effects, making it a great addition to this tea. Together, these two herbs can help reduce fever and alleviate other symptoms associated with seasonal illnesses.

I. FLU: CHAMOMILE AND YARROW HERBAL TEA

Ingredients:

- 1 tablespoon dried chamomile flowers

- 1 tablespoon dried yarrow flowers

- 2 cups water

- Honey (optional)

Instructions:

- In a small pot, bring the water to a boil.

- Add the chamomile and yarrow flowers to the pot and reduce the heat to a simmer.

- Cover the pot and let the herbs simmer for 10-15 minutes.

- After the tea has simmered, strain the liquid into a cup.

- Add honey to taste, if desired.

- Enjoy your Chamomile and Yarrow herbal tea!

Note: Both chamomile and yarrow have been used for centuries for their medicinal properties. Chamomile is known for its calming effects on the body, while yarrow has anti- inflammatory and antibacterial properties that can help boost the immune system. Together, these herbs create a powerful and delicious tea that can help soothe flu symptoms and support overall health.

II. Sore Throat: Thyme and Orange Infusion

Ingredients:

- 1 tablespoon fresh thyme leaves

- 1 orange

- 2 cups water

- 1 tablespoon honey (optional)

Instructions:

- Rinse the thyme leaves and chop them finely.

- Peel the orange and cut the peel into thin strips.

- In a small pot, add the water, thyme, and orange peel.

- Bring the mixture to a boil over medium-high heat.

- Reduce the heat to low and let the mixture simmer for 10 minutes.

- Remove the pot from the heat and strain the liquid into a mug.

- Add honey to taste, if desired.

- Sip the warm infusion slowly to soothe your sore throat.

Note: This infusion can be stored in the refrigerator for up to 2 days. Simply reheat the mixture before drinking. It is a natural and effective remedy for sore throat that can provide relief from discomfort and inflammation.

III. Allergies: Liquor Ice and Nettle Infusion

Ingredients:

- 1 tablespoon of dried liquorice root

- 1 tablespoon of dried nettle leaves

- 4 cups of water

- Honey or lemon (optional)

Instructions:

- In a pot, bring the water to a boil.

- Add the dried liquorice root and nettle leaves to the boiling water.

- Reduce heat to low and let the herbs steep for 10-15 minutes.

- Strain the infusion into a cup.

- Add honey or lemon to taste, if desired.

- Enjoy the infusion while it's warm.

Note: Liquorice root has been used for centuries in traditional medicine for its anti- inflammatory properties. It contains a compound called glycyrrhizin that has been shown to reduce inflammation and soothe sore throats. Additionally, liquorice root may also help reduce the symptoms of allergies, such as congestion and coughing.

IV. Cough: Thyme Ivy infusion

Ingredients:

- 1 tablespoon dried thyme leaves

- 1 tablespoon dried ivy leaves

- 2 cups of water

- 1 tablespoon honey (optional)

Instructions:

- Bring 2 cups of water to a boil in a small saucepan.

- Add 1 tablespoon each of dried thyme and ivy leaves to the boiling water.

- Reduce the heat to low, cover the saucepan and let it simmer for about 15-20 minutes.

- Remove the saucepan from the heat and let it cool for 5 minutes.

- Strain the infusion through a fine mesh strainer or cheesecloth into a teapot or cup.

- Add honey to taste (optional).

- Drink the thyme ivy infusion warm, up to three times a day.

Note: Thyme has natural antitussive (cough suppressant) properties that can help relieve coughing. Ivy has expectorant properties, which means it can help to thin mucus in the lungs and make it easier to cough up. Together, they make a powerful herbal infusion that can help soothe coughs and improve breathing. Adding honey can help sweeten the tea and provide additional soothing benefits.

Muscle Pains, Neck Pain and Migraine

I. Mallow and Lemon Balm Infusion

Ingredients:

- 1 tablespoon of dried mallow leaves

- 1 tablespoon of dried lemon balm leaves

- 4 cups of water

Instructions:

- Boil the water in a pot.

- Add the dried mallow leaves and lemon balm leaves to the boiling water.

- Reduce the heat and let the herbs steep for about 10-15 minutes.

- Strain the infusion using a fine mesh strainer or cheesecloth.

- You can drink the infusion hot or cold. Add honey or lemon to taste, if desired.

- You can drink up to three cups of this infusion per day, preferably after meals.

Note: If you are pregnant, breastfeeding, or taking any medication, consult your healthcare provider before consuming this infusion. Mallow contains high levels of mucilage, which can help soothe inflammation and irritation in the body. Lemon balm, on the other hand, has been traditionally used to calm the nervous system and reduce anxiety. Together, these herbs can help reduce muscle pains, neck pain and migraine by reducing inflammation and promoting relaxation.

II. Herbal Tea with Valerian and Lemon Balm

Ingredients:

- 1 tsp dried valerian root

- 1 tsp dried lemon balm leaves

- 1 cup of water

- Honey (optional)

Instructions:

- Boil the water in a small pot or kettle.

- Add the dried valerian root and lemon balm leaves to a tea infuser or tea bag.

- Place the tea infuser or tea bag in a cup.

- Pour the hot water over the tea infuser or tea bag in the cup.

- Cover the cup and let the tea steep for 10-15 minutes.

- Remove the tea infuser or tea bag from the cup.

- If desired, add honey to taste.

- Enjoy your herbal tea while it's still warm.

Note: Valerian can cause drowsiness, so it's recommended to consume this tea before bed or when you have time to rest. If you're pregnant or breastfeeding, it's best to avoid valerian. Also, consult with a healthcare professional before consuming any herbal remedy, especially if you're taking any medications.

III. Devil's Claw Brew

Ingredients:

- 1 tablespoon of Devil's Claw root powder

- 1 tsp of ginger root powder

- 2 cups of water

- 1 tablespoon of honey (optional)

Instructions:

- Bring 2 cups of water to a boil in a small pot.

- Add 1 tablespoon of Devil's Claw root powder and 1 tsp of ginger root powder to the boiling water.

- Reduce heat and let the mixture simmer for 15-20 minutes.

- Strain the mixture into a mug.

- Add honey to taste if desired.

- Enjoy the warm brew for relief from neck pain and migraines.

Note: Devil's Claw is a natural anti-inflammatory herb that has been used for centuries to relieve pain and discomfort. Ginger also has anti-inflammatory properties and can help with nausea which is sometimes associated with migraines.

Myalgias, Contractures, Strains

PEPPER AND PINEAPPLE INFUSION

Ingredients:

- 1/2 cup fresh pineapple chunks

- 1/4 tsp black pepper

- 1 tsp honey

- 2 cups water

Instructions:

- Add the pineapple chunks to a small saucepan and mash them lightly with a fork to release the juice.

- Add the black pepper and honey to the saucepan and pour in the water.

- Heat the mixture over medium heat until it comes to a boil.

- Reduce the heat to low and let the infusion simmer for 10-15 minutes.

- Strain the mixture through a fine mesh strainer into a cup or mug.

- Let the infusion cool for a few minutes before enjoying.

Note: This unique infusion of pineapple and black pepper offers several health benefits. Pineapple contains an enzyme called bromelain, which has anti-inflammatory properties and may help reduce inflammation associated with conditions like arthritis and asthma. Black pepper is also known to have anti-inflammatory properties and may help relieve pain associated with conditions like osteoarthritis.

II. Orange Blossom and Passion Flower Herbal Tea

Ingredients:

- 2 tbsp dried passion flower

- 2 tbsp dried orange blossom

- 4 cups water

- Honey (optional)

Instructions:

- In a medium-sized pot, bring 4 cups of water to a boil.

- Add 2 tbsp of dried passion flower and 2 tbsp of dried orange blossom to the pot.

- Reduce the heat to low and let the mixture simmer for 5-7 minutes.

- Remove the pot from the heat and let the mixture steep for an additional 5-10 minutes.

- Strain the tea into a cup and add honey to taste if desired.

- Enjoy your soothing and relaxing Orange Blossom and Passion Flower Herbal Tea.

Note: Orange blossom and passion flower are both known for their relaxing and soothing properties, making them ideal for relieving muscle pain, contractures, and strains. Passion flower contains compounds that have a calming effect on the body, helping to reduce muscle tension and alleviate pain. Orange blossom is rich in flavonoids and antioxidants, which help to reduce inflammation and promote healing. This herbal tea can also help to reduce anxiety and promote restful sleep, making it a great addition to your evening routine.

III. Coconut and Cherry Herbal Tea

Ingredients:

- 1 cup of dried cherries

- 1/2 cup of dried coconut flakes

- 4 cups of water

Instructions:

- In a medium-sized pot, bring the water to a boil.

- Once the water is boiling, add the dried cherries and coconut flakes to the pot.

- Reduce the heat to low and allow the mixture to simmer for 10-15 minutes.

- After 10-15 minutes, turn off the heat and let the mixture cool for a few minutes.

- Strain the mixture into a large bowl, removing any solid pieces.

- Pour the tea into a teapot or individual cups and enjoy!

Note: Both cherries and coconut have anti-inflammatory properties, which can help reduce pain and inflammation associated with myalgias, contractures, and strains. Additionally, the natural sweetness of the cherries and coconut flakes can help mask any bitter taste from the herbs, making this tea a delicious and soothing option for muscle pain.

IV. Grape and Ginger Herbal Tea

Ginger Herbal Tea for Myalgias, Contractures, and Strains

Ingredients:

- 1 cup of seedless grapes

- 1 tbsp grated fresh ginger

- 2 cups of water

- 1 tbsp honey (optional)

Instructions:

- Rinse the grapes and cut them in half.

- In a small pot, add the grapes, grated ginger, and water. Bring the mixture to a boil.

- Reduce the heat and let the mixture simmer for about 15 minutes or until the grapes have softened.

- Use a potato masher or a fork to mash the grapes and release the juice.

- Remove from heat and strain the mixture through a fine mesh strainer or cheesecloth.

- If desired, add honey to sweeten the tea.

- Serve hot and enjoy!

Note: Grape and ginger herbal tea is a great way to soothe muscle pains and inflammation caused by myalgias, contractures, and strains. Grapes are high in antioxidants and anti-inflammatory compounds, while ginger is known for its pain- relieving properties. This tea is also a delicious way to stay hydrated and support overall health.

Bodily Inflammations (Internal or External)

I. Blueberry and Dog Rose Herbal Tea

Ingredients:

- 1 cup of blueberries

- 2 tablespoons of dried dog rose petals

- 1 cinnamon stick

- 4 cups of water

- Honey or lemon (optional)

Instructions:

- Rinse the blueberries and add them to a pot with the dried dog rose petals and cinnamon stick.

- Pour in 4 cups of water and bring the mixture to a boil.

- Once it starts boiling, reduce the heat and let it simmer for 10 minutes.

- Remove from heat and let it cool for a few minutes.

- Strain the mixture into a teapot or individual cups.

- Add honey or lemon, if desired, for added flavor and benefits.

- Serve warm and enjoy!

Note: Blueberries are rich in antioxidants and have anti-inflammatory properties that help to reduce inflammation in the body. Dog rose petals are also known for their anti- inflammatory benefits and are rich in vitamin C, which supports the immune system. Cinnamon adds a touch of warmth and also has anti-inflammatory properties. This tea is a delicious way to soothe bodily inflammations and boost your immune system.

II. ECHINACEA AND GINGER HERBAL TEA

Ingredients:

- 1 tbsp dried echinacea root

- 1 tbsp fresh ginger root, peeled and sliced

- 4 cups of water

- Honey (optional)

Instructions:

- Add the dried echinacea root and fresh ginger slices to a medium-sized pot.

- Pour 4 cups of water into the pot and bring it to a boil over medium-high heat.

- Once the water is boiling, reduce the heat to low and let the tea simmer for 10-15 minutes.

- Remove the pot from the heat and strain the tea into a mug using a fine-mesh strainer.

- Add honey to sweeten the tea if desired.

- Enjoy your echinacea and ginger herbal tea while it's still hot.

Note: Echinacea and ginger herbal tea is a great way to boost your immune system and promote overall wellness. Echinacea has been shown to enhance the immune system by stimulating the production of white blood cells, while ginger is known for its anti- inflammatory and antioxidant properties.

III. MORINGA AND BASIL HERBAL TEA

Write a unique recipe content in the right format on Moringa and basil herbal tea Moringa and Basil Herbal Tea Recipe:

Ingredients:

- 1 cup water

- 1 tsp dried moringa leaves

- 1 tsp fresh basil leaves

- 1 tsp honey

- Lemon slices

Instructions:

- In a small saucepan, bring 1 cup of water to a boil.

- Add the dried moringa leaves and fresh basil leaves to the boiling water and let it steep for 5-7 minutes.

- Remove the saucepan from heat and strain the tea to remove the leaves.

- Add honey to the tea, if desired, and stir well.

- Pour the tea into a mug and add lemon slices, if desired, for added flavor.

Note: Moringa leaves can also be used fresh, but make sure to use the same amount as the recipe calls for dried. Adjust the amount of honey to your taste preference. This herbal tea can be enjoyed hot or cold.

IV. Yarrow and Mandarin Tea

Ingredients:

- 1 tablespoon dried yarrow flowers

- 1 mandarin orange, peeled and sliced

- 3 cups of water

- Honey (optional)

Instructions:

- In a small pot, bring the water to a boil.

- Add the dried yarrow flowers to the pot and let steep for 5-10 minutes.

- Add the sliced mandarin orange to the pot and continue to steep for an additional 2-3 minutes.

- Remove the pot from the heat and strain the tea into a cup.

- If desired, sweeten with honey to taste.

- Serve hot and enjoy the soothing and refreshing flavors of yarrow and mandarin.

Note: Yarrow should be avoided during pregnancy and breastfeeding, and should not be consumed in large quantities. Consult with a healthcare professional before consuming this tea if you have any medical conditions or are taking any medications.

V. Turmeric Tea, Milk and Cardamom

Ingredients:

- 1 cup of water

- 1 tsp turmeric powder

- 1/2 tsp cardamom powder

- 1/2 tsp honey (optional)

- 1/2 cup milk (dairy or non-dairy)

Instructions:

- In a small saucepan, bring 1 cup of water to a boil.

- Add 1 tsp turmeric powder and 1/2 tsp cardamom powder to the boiling water.

- Reduce heat to low and let the mixture simmer for 5-10 minutes.

- Strain the tea into a mug.

- Add 1/2 cup of milk and stir.

- Add honey to taste, if desired.

- Serve hot and enjoy!

Note: Turmeric is known for its anti-inflammatory properties, and adding milk and cardamom can make it more palatable and easier for the body to absorb. This tea can be a great way to incorporate turmeric into your diet and potentially aid in reducing inflammation in the body. The addition of cardamom can also promote digestive health and add a pleasant flavor to the tea.

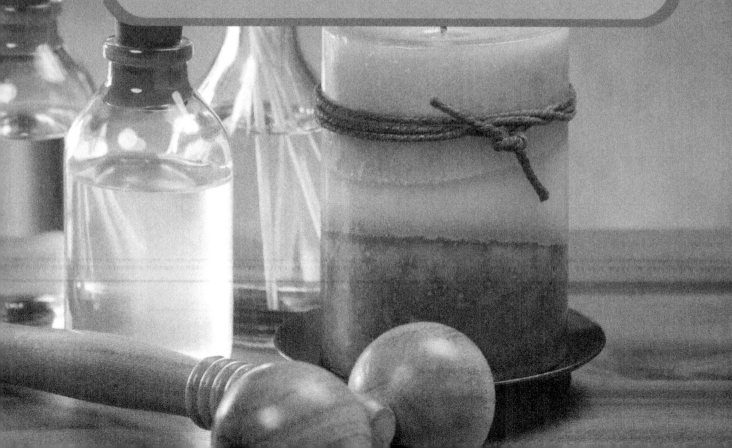

AROMATHERAPY

Chapter 1
WHAT IT IS AND WHERE IT COMES FROM

Aromatherapy is a form of alternative medicine that uses essential oils derived from plants to improve physical, mental, and emotional well-being. It is an ancient practice that has been used for thousands of years in various cultures around the world.

The origins of aromatherapy can be traced back to ancient civilizations such as Egypt, India, and China. In Egypt, essential oils were used in the embalming process and were also used for medicinal purposes. The famous Ebers Papyrus, an ancient Egyptian medical text, contains references to the use of essential oils for a variety of health conditions.

In India, aromatherapy was practiced as part of Ayurvedic medicine, which is one of the oldest systems of medicine in the world. Ayurveda uses essential oils to balance the body, mind, and spirit and promote overall well-being. In China, aromatherapy has been used as part of Traditional Chinese Medicine (TCM) for thousands of years. Essential oils are used in TCM to improve the flow of energy in the body and promote healing.

The modern practice of aromatherapy can be attributed to the French chemist Rene- Maurice Gattefosse, who discovered the healing properties of lavender essential oil when he accidentally burned his hand and then immersed it in a vat of lavender oil. He was surprised to find that the burn healed quickly and without scarring, which led him to investigate the properties of essential oils further. Gattefosse went on to publish a book on the therapeutic properties of essential oils, and he coined the term "aromatherapy" to describe the use of essential oils for therapeutic purposes.

The practice of aromatherapy has since evolved and has become increasingly popular in the Western world, where it is used to alleviate a variety of health conditions and promote overall well-being. Today, aromatherapy is used in a variety of settings, including spas, clinics, hospitals, and homes. It is used to treat a range of health conditions, including anxiety, depression, insomnia, pain, and skin conditions, among others. Aromatherapy is also used for relaxation, stress relief, and to promote a sense of calm and well-being.

BENEFITS AND RISKS

Aromatherapy is a holistic approach to health and wellness that uses essential oils derived from plants to promote physical and emotional well-being. While there are many potential benefits to aromatherapy, it is important to understand that there are also risks associated with its use. In this article, we will explore the benefits and risks of aromatherapy in ascending order.

BENEFITS:

- **Improved Mood:** Aromatherapy can help to improve mood and reduce feelings of anxiety and depression. Essential oils such as lavender and chamomile are known for their calming properties and can promote relaxation.

- **Pain Relief:** Certain essential oils, such as peppermint and eucalyptus, have been shown to provide pain relief for headaches, muscle aches, and other types of pain.

- **Improved Sleep:** Aromatherapy can promote relaxation and improve sleep quality. Essential oils such as lavender and bergamot are known for their ability to promote restful sleep.

- **Reduced Inflammation:** Some essential oils, such as frankincense and turmeric, have anti-inflammatory properties and can help to reduce inflammation in the body.

- **Enhanced Immune System:** Aromatherapy can help to enhance the immune system by stimulating the production of white blood cells and improving circulation.

RISKS:

- **Allergic Reactions:** Some people may experience allergic reactions to certain essential oils. It is important to test a small amount of the oil on your skin before using it more extensively.

- **Skin Irritation:** Essential oils can cause skin irritation, especially when used in high concentrations or when applied directly to the skin. It is important to dilute essential oils with a carrier oil before use.

- **Toxicity:** Some essential oils, such as camphor and pennyroyal, can be toxic when ingested. It is important to use essential oils only as directed and to keep them out of reach of children.

- **Interactions with Medications:** Essential oils can interact with certain medications, including blood thinners and antidepressants. It is important to speak with a healthcare provider before using aromatherapy if you are taking any medications.

- **Quality Control:** There is limited regulation of the aromatherapy industry, which can lead to variations in the quality and purity of essential oils. It is important to purchase essential oils from a reputable source and to carefully read the labels and ingredient lists before use.

HOW TO USE IT FOR OUR NEEDS

- **Determine your desired outcome:** The first step in using aromatherapy for your needs is to determine your desired outcome. Do you want to feel relaxed, energized, focused, or something else? Different essential oils have different properties and can help with a variety of conditions, so it's important to choose the right one for your needs.

- **Choose the right essential oil:** Once you have determined your desired outcome, it's time to choose the right essential oil. There are many different essential oils to choose from, each with its own unique properties and benefits. For example, lavender is known for its calming and relaxing properties, while peppermint is energizing and can help with focus and concentration.

- **Decide on your method of application:** There are several ways to apply essential oils, including inhalation, topical application, and ingestion. Inhalation is the most common method and involves using a diffuser or simply inhaling the scent directly from the bottle. The topical application involves diluting the essential oil with a carrier oil and applying it directly to the skin, while ingestion should only be done under the guidance of a qualified aromatherapist.

- **Use the appropriate dosage:** It's important to use the appropriate dosage when using essential oils. The amount of oil needed will vary depending on the desired outcome and the method of application. Always follow the recommended dosage on the bottle or seek guidance from a qualified aromatherapist.

- **Be aware of potential risks:** While essential oils can be very beneficial, it's important to be aware of potential risks. Essential oils are highly concentrated and can be toxic if ingested or applied undiluted to the skin. Some oils can also cause allergic reactions in some people. Always use essential oils with caution and seek guidance from a qualified aromatherapist if you have any concerns.

- **Enjoy the benefits:** When used safely and appropriately, aromatherapy can provide a wide range of benefits, including stress relief, improved sleep, pain relief, and more. Experiment with different oils and methods of application to find what works best for you and enjoy the many benefits of aromatherapy.

Chapter 2

RECIPES WITH ESSENTIAL OILS

'Regain Serenity' (Lavender, Bergamot, Cedar)

Ingredients:

- 10 drops lavender essential oil

- 10 drops bergamot essential oil

- 10 drops cedar essential oil

- 1 oz carrier oil (such as sweet almond oil or jojoba oil)

Instructions:

- In a clean glass bottle, add the lavender, bergamot, and cedar essential oils.

- Gently swirl the bottle to mix the oils together.

- Add the carrier oil to the bottle, making sure it covers the essential oils.

- Secure the lid and shake well to combine.

- Store the blend in a cool, dark place.

Instructions:

- Apply a small amount of the Regain Serenity blend to the palms of your hands.

- Rub your hands together to warm the oil and release the scent.

- Cup your hands over your nose and mouth and take several deep breaths, inhaling the aroma.

- Repeat as often as needed throughout the day to help promote feelings of calm and relaxation.

Note: This blend is for external use only. Do not ingest. If irritation occurs, discontinue use. Always perform a patch test before using any essential oil blend on your skin.

'Start Over' (Mandarin, Sage, Mint)

Ingredients:

- 1 tbsp dried mandarin peel

- 1 tbsp dried sage leaves

- 1 tbsp dried peppermint leaves

Instructions:

- Combine all the dried ingredients in a bowl and mix well.

- Place the mixture into a tea infuser or a muslin tea bag.

- Boil 2 cups of water in a saucepan and remove from heat.

- Place the tea infuser or tea bag into the hot water and let it steep for 5-10 minutes.

- Remove the tea infuser or tea bag from the water and discard the herbs.

- Serve hot and enjoy the refreshing aroma and taste of the 'Start Over' blend.

Note: The combination of mandarin, sage, and mint provides a refreshing and uplifting scent that can help to promote mental clarity, boost concentration, and reduce stress and anxiety. Mandarin is known for its calming and soothing properties, while sage is often used to enhance memory and focus. Peppermint is a natural stimulant that can help to improve alertness and reduce fatigue. Drinking this herbal blend regularly can help to improve your overall well-being and give you a fresh start to your day.

'For a good awakening ' (Grapefruit, Peppermint)

Ingredients:

- 5 drops of grapefruit essential oil

- 3 drops of peppermint essential oil

- 1 oz of distilled water

- A small spray bottle

Instructions:

- Fill a small spray bottle with 1 oz of distilled water.

- Add 5 drops of grapefruit essential oil and 3 drops of peppermint essential oil to the bottle.

- Shake the bottle vigorously to mix the oils and water together.

- Spray the mist in the air, on your pillow or around your room to help wake you up and start your day feeling energized.

Note: Alternatively, you can also use this blend in a diffuser or mix it with a carrier oil like coconut or almond oil to use as a body oil or massage oil to help invigorate your senses and improve your mood. Just be sure to do a patch test first and consult with a healthcare provider if you have any allergies or medical conditions.

'Be romantic' (Damascena rose, Mandarin, Sweet orange, Sandalwood)

Ingredients:

- 2 drops Damascena rose essential oil

- 2 drops Mandarin essential oil

- 2 drops sweet orange essential oil

- 2 drops Sandalwood essential oil

- 1 oz carrier oil (such as jojoba or almond oil)

Instructions:

- Mix the essential oils and carrier oil together in a small glass bottle.

- Close the bottle and shake well to blend the oils.

- Apply a small amount of the mixture to the wrists, neck, and chest area.

- Inhale deeply and enjoy the romantic and relaxing scent.

Note: Damascena rose essential oil is known for its romantic and aphrodisiac properties, helping to promote relaxation and calmness. Mandarin essential oil can help ease tension and anxiety, promoting a calm and relaxed state of mind. Sweet orange essential oil has a bright and uplifting scent, promoting positivity and joy. Sandalwood essential oil has a grounding and calming effect, promoting relaxation and inner peace.

Be romantic' (Damascena rose, Mandarin, Sweet orange, Sandalwood)
'Antidepressant remedy' (Grapefruit, Neroli)

Ingredients:

- 5 drops grapefruit essential oil

- 5 drops neroli essential oil

- 10 ml carrier oil (such as sweet almond or jojoba oil)

- A small glass bottle with a lid

Instructions:

- Begin by adding 5 drops of grapefruit essential oil and 5 drops of neroli essential oil to the small glass bottle.

- Pour in 10 ml of carrier oil of your choice.

- Secure the lid on the bottle and shake gently to mix the oils together.

- Store the bottle in a cool, dark place away from direct sunlight or heat.

- To use, add a few drops of the blend to a diffuser, oil burner or inhaler and inhale deeply for a few minutes.

- Apply the blend topically to your temples, wrists, or chest.

Note: Remember to perform a patch test before applying the blend directly to your skin. The uplifting aroma of grapefruit and the calming, grounding scent of neroli combine to create a blend that can help alleviate the symptoms of depression and promote emotional balance. This blend can also be effective in reducing anxiety, stress, and tension.

Bonus Guide

YOUR GARDEN AT HOME

HOW TO GROW PLANTS AND MEDICINAL HERBS AT HOME

It's a terrific way to add some greenery to your home and to have quick access to fresh herbs for cooking or medicinal purposes by growing plants and medicinal herbs in your own home. You can grow a wide variety of plants at home, including potted aromatic plants, outdoor plants, and medicinal herbs. Here are some pointers and tricks to get you going:

- **Aromatic Plants in Pots:**

Because they require little maintenance and can be utilized in cooking, aromatherapy, or just for their pleasant perfume, aromatic plants are an excellent choice for growing in pots. Make sure the pot you select has adequate drainage holes and is the proper size for your plant. Any container can be used as long as it contains drainage holes. Using a saucer to collect extra water is another smart move. To promote drainage, choose a potting mixture with good drainage qualities and add some perlite or coarse sand to the mixture. Put the pot somewhere sunny, ideally close to a window that receives at least six hours of direct sunlight each day, as aromatic plants require sunlight to grow. Pruning your plant on a regular basis will keep it bushy and healthy.

- **Choosing the Right Pot:**

Think about the size of the plant, the root system, and the setting before selecting a pot for your plants. Select plant containers for indoor plants that go with your decor and enhance the space. Choose sturdy, weather-resistant pots for outdoor plants. Because they are porous and promote airflow, terracotta pots are a popular choice for outdoor plants. Plastic pots are cheap, lightweight, and available in a wide range of hues and patterns. Ceramic pots are fashionable and available in a wide range of sizes and forms, but they may also be bulky and delicate.

- **The Needs of Outdoor Plants:**

Due to their exposure to the weather and higher maintenance needs, outdoor plants have different requirements than indoor plants. Consider the weather and the amount of sunlight the plants will receive when selecting outside plants. While some plants like full or partial shade, others do well in direct sunlight. Regularly water your outdoor plants, especially in the summer when it's hot and dry. Use fertilizer made exclusively for outdoor plants and adhere to the directions on the container. To keep your outside plants healthy and bushy, prune them frequently.

- **Choosing the Right Soil for Your Medicinal Garden:**

It's crucial to select the proper soil while growing medicinal herbs in order for your plants to grow robustly and healthily. Pick a potting mix with strong drainage qualities since medicinal herbs prefer well-draining soil. To increase drainage, you can also add some perlite or coarse sand to the mixture. Given that toxins and chemicals might have an impact on the quality of your herbs, it is crucial to select soil that is free of them.

- **When to Sow:**

The sort of plant you are growing and the climate where you live will determine the optimal time to plant seeds for your medicinal garden. While some plants should be started indoors and moved outside in the summer, others can be seeded immediately in the ground in the spring. It's crucial to read the directions on the seed packaging and do your homework on the particular requirements of your plants.

- **Home Garden: How to Get Good Results:**

Making the correct choices for your home garden's plants, soil, and atmosphere is crucial for success. Pick plants that will flourish in your environment and receive the necessary quantity of sunshine. Use a high-quality potting mix with excellent drainage and nutritional content. Make sure to give your plants regular watering and fertilize them using a fertilizer that is made especially for them. To keep your plants healthy and bushy, prune them frequently.

• The Utility of Spices for Your Dishes:

Many foods require the use of spices since they enhance flavor, scent, and health. A wonderful way to guarantee that your spices are both fresh and free of pesticides and chemicals is to grow them yourself at home. Basil, thyme, rosemary, mint, and cilantro are a few well-known spices that you may cultivate in your own backyard. You can cultivate these in pots or in a tiny herb garden. Spices should be harvested in the morning when the oils are at their highest concentration for the finest flavor and scent. To use your spices later in the year, you may also dry them.

In conclusion, home gardening is a satisfying and enjoyable activity that has a lot of potential advantages. Your plants will grow well and robustly if you choose the appropriate containers, soil, and surroundings. Maintaining and pruning your plants on a regular basis will keep them robust and bushy, and picking your herbs at the correct time will guarantee that they are at their most fragrant and aromatic. A home garden can be a wonderful addition to any living area, whether you are growing herbs for cooking or for their health benefits.

Index

Printed in Great Britain
by Amazon